# Sm... Medical Differential Diagnosis

## A BOOK OF LISTS

Fourth Edition

# Small Animal Medical Differential Diagnosis

## A BOOK OF LISTS

## MARK S. THOMPSON, DVM

Diplomate, American Board of Veterinary Practitioners
Certified in Canine/Feline Practice
Brevard Animal Hospital
Brevard, North Carolina

ELSEVIER

Elsevier
3251 Riverport Lane
St. Louis, Missouri 63043

Small Animal Medical Differential Diagnosis,
FOURTH EDITION

**ISBN:** 978-0-323-87590-5

Previous editions copyrighted 2018, 2014, and 2007.

*Content Strategist*: Jennifer Catando
*Senior Content Development Specialist*: Ambika Kapoor
*Publishing Services Manager*: Deepthi Unni
*Project Manager*: Sindhuraj Thulasingam
*Design Direction*: Brian Salisbury

Printed in India

Last digit is the print number:   9   8   7   6   5   4   3   2   1

*In memory of my father, Jon Hobert Thompson, from whom I got my work ethic and my sense of humor. Both attributes have helped me to develop and to enjoy my career as a veterinarian.*

Who knew that this little book of lists would do well enough to be revised again and again? But veterinary medical literature marches on; changing, expanding, and revising itself, as we all know it should. So here we go again; the fourth edition of *Small Animal Medical Differential Diagnosis: A Book of Lists*. The lists of the third edition have been updated and about twenty new lists have been added. As before, the goal was to provide a quick, concise, and practical reference to differential diagnosis, etiology, laboratory values, and classification of clinical signs and medical disorders in dogs and cats. And as before, nearly all the lists required additions, subtractions, or sometimes complete reorganization. Once again, this text will be a pocket-sized rapid reference or an electronic application. Its greatest value will be to aid the clinician in making reliable, on-the-scene decisions and to allow veterinary students and interns to more fully participate in clinical rounds with their instructors. It will also be used by the more seasoned practitioner to come up with those more esoteric differentials that we sometimes forget to include in our list of potential diagnoses.

The lists in this book have been compiled from comprehensive veterinary references published by Elsevier, especially:

Ettinger, Feldman, and Côté: Textbook of Veterinary Internal Medicine, 8th ed.

Nelson and Couto: Small Animal Internal Medicine, 6th ed.

Cohn and Côté: Clinical Veterinary Advisor, 4th ed.

Also consulted for information were:

Johnston and Tobias: Veterinary Surgery, Small Animal, 2nd ed.

Valenciano and Cowell: Cowell and Tyler's Diagnostic Cytology and Hematology, 5th ed.

Withrow and MacEwen: Small Animal Clinical Oncology, 6th ed.

Mattoon, Sellon, and Berry: Small Animal Diagnostic Ultrasound, 4th ed.

The reader is encouraged to consult these and other texts for more detailed information.

## About the Book

As with the first three editions, the lists are divided into three parts and serve as a concise guide to the differential diagnosis, etiology, laboratory abnormalities, and classification of clinical signs and medical disorders in dogs and cats. Part One contains lists based on clinical signs that may be identified by the clinician. Part Two approaches the differential diagnosis from a systems perspective. Fifteen body systems are represented. Additionally, there is a section in Part Two that features lists about focused assessment with sonography for trauma (FAST) ultrasound. Point-of-care, rapid ultrasound techniques are used as an extension of the physical exam in ill or injured patients and as such, FAST ultrasound has become an integral skill in the establishment of a differential diagnosis. Part Three is once again a quick reference of laboratory tests and gives typical normal ranges and differential diagnoses based on test results. Overall, the book comprises approximately 450 lists, 20 of which are new to this edition. In all lists, an attempt has been made to prioritize them from least common to most common.

## Acknowledgments

I wish to thank my fellow veterinarians at Brevard Animal Hospital: Dr. Lindsay Batson, Dr. Heather Garland, Dr. Lucia Fleischmann, and Dr. Jamilea Van Hemel. They were a sounding board for ideas and helped me discover deficiencies in the first three editions. In addition, our discussions about cases helped me determine new lists that needed to be generated.

PART ONE

# Clinical Signs Approach to Differential Diagnosis, *1*

# CLINICAL SIGNS APPROACH TO DIFFERENTIAL DIAGNOSIS

## Abdominal Distension

### Organomegaly

Hepatomegaly (infiltrative, inflammatory, lipidosis, neoplasia)

Splenomegaly (infiltrative, inflammatory, neoplasia, hematoma)

Renomegaly (neoplasia, infiltrative)

Miscellaneous neoplasia (gastrointestinal [GI] tract, ovaries, uterus, pancreas, prostate, adrenal glands)

Generalized neoplasia (carcinomatosis, lymphosarcoma)

Granuloma (pythiosis, aspergillosis)

Pregnancy

Prostatomegaly

Reactive lymphadenopathy

### Fluid

#### CONTAINED IN ORGANS

Congestion resulting from splenic torsion or volvulus, or hepatic congestion from right-sided heart failure

Cysts (paraprostatic, perinephric, hepatic)

Hydronephrosis

Distended urinary bladder

Obstruction of intestines or stomach

Ileus

Pyometra

#### FREE FLUID IN ABDOMEN

Transudate (portal hypertension, right-sided heart failure, hypoproteinemia secondary to protein-losing enteropathy, protein-losing nephropathy, or hepatic failure)

Modified transudate (neoplasia, postsinusoidal portal hypertension, right-sided heart failure, heartworm-related caval syndrome, liver disease)

Exudate (pancreatitis, feline infectious peritonitis [FIP], urine, bile, neoplasia, bowel perforation, foreign body)

Chyle (trauma, neoplasia, infection, right-sided heart failure)

Blood (coagulopathy, trauma, neoplasia)

### Gas

#### CONTAINED IN ORGANS

Gastric dilatation/volvulus

Intestines secondary to obstruction

Parenchymal organs infected with gas-producing bacteria (emphysematous gallbladder or urinary bladder)

**FREE IN ABDOMEN**
Iatrogenic (after laparoscopy, laparotomy)
Rupture of GI tract or uterus

## Fat

Obesity/lipoma

## Weakened Abdominal Musculature

Hyperadrenocorticism

## Feces

Obstipation/megacolon

### Abdominal Effusions and Ascites

## Transudate (<1000 Cells, <2.5 Total Solids, <1.017 Specific Gravity)

**PORTAL HYPERTENSION**
Presinusoidal or sinusoidal liver disease
Right-sided heart failure

**HYPOALBUMINEMIA (SEE ALBUMIN, P. 328)**
Liver failure
Protein-losing enteropathy

**GLOMERULOPATHY**

## Modified Transudate (>1000 but <10,000 Cells, 2.5–5.0 Total Solids, <1.025 Specific Gravity)

**POSTSINUSOIDAL PORTAL HYPERTENSION**

**RIGHT-SIDED HEART FAILURE**
Heartworm-related caval syndrome
Liver disease

**NEOPLASIA**

## Increased Hydrostatic Pressure

## Vasculitis

## Exudate (>5000 Cells, >3.0 Total Solids, >1.025 Specific Gravity)

**NONSEPTIC**
Pancreatitis
FIP
Urine
Bile
Neoplasia (mesothelioma, lymphoma, carcinomatosis, any mass that causes lymphatic or vascular obstruction)

**SEPTIC**
Bowel perforation
Foreign body

## Chyle

Trauma
Neoplasia
Infection
Right-sided heart failure

## Blood

Coagulopathy
Trauma
Neoplasia (hemangiosarcoma, hepatocellular carcinoma)
Iatrogenic (postsurgical)

## Abortion

### Risk Factors

Malnutrition
Advanced maternal age
Previous loss of pregnancy (e.g. recurrent hypoluteoidism)
Endocrine (hypothyroidism, hyperadrenocorticism, diabetes mellitus, hypoluteioidism)
Infectious (*Brucella, Streptococcus, Escherichia coli, Listeria, Salmonella, Chlamydia, Mycoplasma, Leptospira, Campylobacter*, canine herpesvirus 1, parvovirus, bluetongue virus, canine distemper virus, canine adenovirus, *Leishmania, Toxoplasma, Borrelia, Ehrlichia, Anaplasma*)
Drugs (e.g., corticosteroids, itraconazole, griseofulvin)
Toxins (e. g., plant toxins, insecticides)

## Abdominal Pain, Acute

### Gastrointestinal System

GI ulceration
Foreign body
Gastric dilation/volvulus
Gastroenteritis
Obstipation
Colitis
Neoplasia
Adhesions
Intestinal ischemia
Intestinal spasm
Intussusception
Flatulence

## Urogenital System

Lower urinary tract infection
Lower urinary tract obstruction
Nonseptic cystitis (idiopathic cystitis—cats)
Prostatitis/prostatic neoplasia
Uroliths/renoliths/ureterolith
Pyelonephritis
Neoplasm
Metritis
Pyometra/uterine rupture
Uterine torsion (rare)
Testicular torsion
Mastitis
Dystocia
Ovarian cyst

## Pancreatitis

## Spleen

Rupture
Neoplasm
Infection
Torsion

## Peritoneum

Peritonitis
• Septic
• Nonseptic (e.g., uroabdomen)
Adhesions
Mesenteric neoplasia, volvulus, inflammation

## Hepatobiliary

Hepatitis
Hepatic abscess
Hepatic trauma, rupture
Hepatobiliary neoplasia
Cholelithiasis or cholecystitis
Cholangiohepatitis

## Musculoskeletal

Fractures
Intervertebral disk disease
Discospondylitis
Abscess
Strangulated hernia

## Miscellaneous

Adrenalitis (associated with hypoadrenocorticism)

Heavy metal intoxication
Vasculopathy
- Rocky Mountain spotted fever
- Infarct
Autonomic (abdominal) epilepsy
Iatrogenic
- Misoprostol
- Bethanechol
- Postoperative pain

## Abuse

### Historical Signs of Abuse

Animal show fear of owner, happier away from owner
Behavior of presenting person (embarrassed, aggressive, implausible, discomfited, lack of concern for animal)
Discrepant history (changing story, differing history from person to person)
Family violence known or suspected
Lack of history of any accident to explain the injury
Injury too severe to fit the history
Particular person implicated (child, partner, self-implication)
Previous unexplained injury or death of another pet in the same home
Repetitive injury (more than one presentation, differing ages of injuries/fractures identified)

### Physical Signs of Abuse

Fractures (skull, ribs, femur most common)
Internal injury: rupture of internal organs such as liver, spleen, kidney, urinary bladder.
Intrapulmonary hemorrhage
Superficial bruising (head, thorax, abdomen, limbs, scleral/conjunctival hemorrhage), especially over bony prominences such as ribs or vertebrae
Sexual abuse injuries involving genitalia or anal area. Both sexes may be abused

## Acidosis, Metabolic

### Increased Anion Gap

Diabetic ketoacidosis
Uremic acidosis
Lactic acidosis

Toxicants (ethylene glycol, salicylates, paraldehyde, methanol)

## Normal Anion Gap

Diarrhea
Renal tubular acidosis
Hypoadrenocorticism
Carbonic anhydrase inhibitors (e.g., acetazolamide)
Ammonium chloride
Cationic amino acids
Posthypocapnic metabolic acidosis
Dilutional (e.g., rapid administration of saline)

## Acidosis, Respiratory

## Airway Obstruction

Collapsing trachea
Asthma
Aspiration (foreign body, vomitus)
Mass (neoplasia, abscess)
Obstructed endotracheal tube
Brachycephalic airway syndrome
Laryngeal paralysis, laryngospasm
Bronchiectasis

## Pulmonary and Small Airway Disease

Pulmonary edema
Pneumonia
Pulmonary thromboembolism
Diffuse metastatic disease
Acute respiratory distress syndrome
Asthma
Pulmonary fibrosis
Smoke inhalation
Bronchiectasis

## Respiratory Center Depression

Neurologic disease (brain stem, high cervical spinal cord lesion)
Drugs (narcotics, sedatives, barbiturates, inhalation anesthetics)

## Impaired Alveolar Ventilation

Cardiopulmonary arrest
Heat stroke
Malignant hyperthermia

## Neuromuscular Defects

Tick paralysis
Myasthenia gravis
Polyradiculoneuritis
Polymyositis
Botulism
Tetanus
Hypokalemic myopathy in cats
Hypokalemic periodic paralysis in Burmese cats
Drugs (neuromuscular blocking agents, aminoglycosides, organophosphates)

## Restrictive Extrapulmonary Disorders

Diaphragmatic hernia
Pleural space disease
Chest wall trauma/flail chest

## Marked Obesity (Pickwickian Syndrome)

## Inadequate Mechanical Ventilation

## Aggressive Behavior

### Cats

#### PATHOPHYSIOLOGIC CAUSES OF FELINE AGGRESSION

Rabies
Toxoplasmosis
Hyperthyroidism
Seizures (epilepsy, central nervous system [CNS] inflammation)
Paradoxical effects of therapeutic drugs (e.g., benzodiazepines)
Toxins (side effects)
Cognitive dysfunction
Brain neoplasia

#### SPECIES-TYPICAL PATTERNS OF FELINE AGGRESSION TOWARD HUMANS

Defensive response when threatened, (may freeze, retreat, climb, or hide, but aggression eventually becomes an option), worse in feral and cats not sensitized to people between 2–7 weeks of age
Play/predatory/attention-seeking response
Aggression as a response to frustration (also known as redirected aggression)

Aggression that arises as a result of disease processes (see Pathophysiologic Causes of Feline Aggression earlier)

Interspecies aggression (either fear induced or territorial/ resource guarding)

## Dogs

### PATHOPHYSIOLOGIC CAUSES OF CANINE AGGRESSION

Rabies

Seizure activity

Intracranial neoplasia

Cerebral hypoxia

Neuroendocrine disturbances

### SPECIES-TYPICAL PATTERNS OF CANINE AGGRESSION

Fear related

Conflict related

Resource guarding

Territorial/protective

Intraspecific (intradog)

Redirected

Predatory

Pain/medical/irritable

Play

Maternal/hormonal

Idiopathic

## Alkalosis, Metabolic

### Chlorine Responsive

Vomiting of stomach contents

Diuretic therapy

Posthypercapnia

### Chlorine Resistant

Hyperadrenocorticism

Primary hyperaldosteronism

### Alkali Administration

Oral sodium bicarbonate or other organic anion (e.g., lactate, citrate, gluconate, acetate)

Oral cation exchange resin with nonabsorbable alkali (phosphate binder)

### Miscellaneous

Severe potassium or magnesium deficiency

Refeeding after fasting

High-dose penicillin therapy

## Alkalosis, Respiratory

### Hypoxemia

Congestive heart failure
Severe anemia
Right-to-left shunting
Decreased cardiac output
Decreased $PiO_2$ (high altitude)
Severe hypotension
Ventilation-perfusion mismatch
- Pneumonia
- Pulmonary thromboembolism
- Pulmonary edema
- Pulmonary thrombosis
- Acute pulmonary distress syndrome (ARDS)

### Pulmonary Disease (Stimulation of Stretch/Nociceptors Independent of Hypoxemia)

Pneumonia
Pulmonary edema
ARDS
Pulmonary thromboembolism
Interstitial lung disease

### Centrally Mediated Hyperventilation

Liver disease
Gram-negative sepsis
Drugs: salicylate intoxication, progesterone (pregnancy), xanthines (e.g., aminophylline)
Recovery from metabolic acidosis
Central neurologic disease
- Trauma
- Neoplasia
- Infection
- Inflammation
- Cerebrospinal accident
Exercise
Heatstroke

### Overzealous mechanical ventilation

### Situations causing pain, fear, or anxiety

## Alopecia

### Inflammatory Alopecia

**TRAUMATIC**
Allergy (flea, atopy, food)

Parasitic dermatitis (fleas, scabies, *Cheyletiella* spp., lice, chiggers, etc.)

### INFECTIOUS
Pyoderma
Demodicosis
Dermatophytosis
Viral
Leishmaniasis
*Malassezia* spp.

### IMMUNE-MEDIATED
Sebaceous adenitis
Superficial pemphigus
Alopecia areata
Erythema multiforme
Systemic lupus erythematosus (SLE), discoid lupus erythematosus (DLE)
Epitheliotropic lymphoma
Vasculitis
Postrabies vaccination panniculitis and alopecia

### ATROPHIC
Dermatomyositis
Cutaneous vasculitis
Postvaccinal alopecia
Lymphocytic mural folliculitis
Paraneoplastic exfoliative dermatitis
Pseudopelade

## Noninflammatory Alopecia

### HORMONAL
Hyperadrenocorticism
Iatrogenic Cushing syndrome
Hypothyroidism
Sex hormone imbalance
Alopecia X
Hyperthyroidism (cat)

### CANINE AND FELINE PINNAL ALOPECIA

### CANINE PATTERN BALDNESS (ESP. BOSTON TERRIER, DACHSHUND)

### CANINE FOLLICULAR DYSPLASIA
Trichorrhexis nodosa
Pili torti
Color dilution alopecia
Black hair follicular dysplasia

Canine flank alopecia
Anagen and telogen effluvium

### FELINE CONGENITAL/HEREDITARY
Alopecia universalis (Sphinx)
Congenital hypotrichosis
Hair shaft dysplasia (Abyssinian)
Follicular dysplasia (Cornish Rex)
Pili torti

### OTHER
Anagen effluvium
Telogen defluxion
Paraneoplastic alopecia
Cyclic follicular dysplasia (seasonal flank alopecia)
Postclipping alopecia
Cicatricial alopecia
Feline preauricular alopecia
Feline acquired symmetric alopecia
Psychogenic alopecia

## Amyloidosis

### Infectious

Bacterial
- Polynephritis
- Pyometra
- Pyoderma
- Other chronic bacterial infections

Protozoal
- Hepatozoonosis
- Leishmaniasis

Parasitic
- Dirofilariasis

Fungal
- Blastomycosis
- Coccidioidomycosis

### Inflammatory

- Dermatitis, chronic
- Dermatomyositis
- Inflammatory bowel disease
- Pancreatitis
- Periodontal disease
- Polyarthritis
- Systemic lupus erythematosus

## Neoplastic

- Lymphoma
- Myeloma
- Other neoplasia

## Familial

- Shar-Pei
- Abyssinian cat
- Siamese cat

## Miscellaneous

- Hyperlipidemia
- Congenital C3 deficiency
- Chronic insulin infusion
- Cyclic hematopoiesis of gray Collies

## Idiopathic

## Anaphylaxis

## Venoms

Insects of Hymenoptera order (bees, hornets, ants)
Spiders (brown recluse, black widow)
Snakes (rattlesnakes, copperheads, water moccasins)
Lizards (Gila monster, Mexican beaded lizard)

## Drugs

Antibiotics (penicillins, sulfonamides, lincomycin, cephalosporins, aminoglycosides, tetracyclines, chloramphenicol, polymyxin B)
Vaccines
Allergen extracts
Blood products
Parasiticides (dichlorophen, levamisole, piperazine, dichlorvos, diethylcarbamazine, thiacetarsamide)
Anesthetics/sedatives (acepromazine, ketamine, barbiturates, lidocaine, bupivacaine, narcotics, diazepam)
Nonsteroidal antiinflammatory drugs (NSAIDs)
Hormones (insulin, corticotropin, vasopressin, parathyroid hormone, glucocorticoids)
Aminophylline
Chemotherapeutics (doxorubicin, L-asparaginase, docetaxel, paclitaxel, etoposide)
Iodinated contrast media
Neostigmine
Amphotericin B

Enzymes (trypsin, chymotrypsin)
Vitamins (vitamin K, thiamine, folic acid)
Dextrans and gelatins
Calcium disodium edetate

## Foods

Milk, egg white, shellfish, legumes, citrus fruits, chocolate,
grains

## Physical Factors

Cold, heat, exercise

# Anorexia

## Primary Anorexia

Disinterest in eating; primary disease of appetite or satiety
centers, rare

## Secondary Anorexia (Common With Virtually Any Systemic Disease)

Associated with nausea (GI inflammation, ileus, delayed
gastric emptying, vestibular disease, drug-induced nausea,
food aversion)

## Pseudoanorexia (Reluctance to Eat)

Retrobulbar abscess
Intraoral masses, foreign bodies
Mandibular fractures/temporomandibular joint disease
Masticatory myositis
Periodontal disease, gingivostomatitis
Salivary mucocele, sialadenitis, salivary tumor
Oropharyngeal dysphagia
Esophageal masses or foreign bodies
Nasal disease
Unpalatable diet
Anosmia

## Behavioral

Social stress or conflict
Anxiety
Loss of companion

# Anuria and Oliguria

## Prerenal Azotemia

Dehydration/hypovolemia

## Acute Renal Failure

One-third of cases are anuric, one-third are oliguric, and one-third are nonoliguric; more likely to be oliguric/anuric with severe renal toxicosis

Toxic: exogenous (drugs, biologic or environmental toxins), endogenous (calcium, pigments)

Infectious: pyelonephritis, leptospirosis, infectious canine hepatitis, borreliosis, sepsis

Ischemia: progression of prerenal azotemia, NSAIDs, vascular disease (avulsion, thrombosis, stenosis), shock, decreased cardiac output, deep anesthesia, extensive surgery, hypothermia, hyperthermia, hyperviscosity (polycythemia vera, multiple myeloma, extensive cutaneous burns, transfusion reaction, disseminated intravascular coagulation [DIC])

Immune-mediated: acute glomerulonephritis, SLE, transplant rejection, vasculitis

Neoplasia: lymphoma

Systemic disease with renal manifestations: Infections (FIP, borreliosis, babesiosis, leishmaniasis, bacterial endocarditis); Pancreatitis; Sepsis; Multiple organ failure; Heart failure; SLE; Hepatorenal disease; Malignant hypertension; Acute hyperphosphatemia (tumor lysis syndrome)

## Postrenal Azotemia

Obstruction (may appear similar to anuria/oliguria)

## Anxiety and Phobias

### Fears and Phobias

Fear: apprehension associated with the presence of an object, individual, or sound; may be normal or abnormal, depending on context

Phobia: quickly developed, immediate, profound abnormal response to a stimulus leading to catatonia or panic

#### PEOPLE

Babies, children, elderly

People in uniform

People who appear different from family members
- Color, height, facial hair

People with disabilities

Men or women, depending on circumstance

### ANIMALS
Same species
Other species

### NOISE
Especially gunshots, fireworks, thunder

### PLACES
Veterinary clinic, grooming facility, kennel
Car, moving vehicle
Crate or specific room
Type of flooring or surface

## Anxiety

### SEPARATION ANXIETY

*Initiators*
Change in owner's routine
Owner returning to school or work
Move to new home
Visit to new environment
After stay in kennel
New baby, new pet, new partner
Medical, cognitive

*Common Features of Separation Anxiety*
Hyperattached to owner
Signs of anxiety as owner leaves
Problems manifest when owner absent or when pet
  unable to gain access to owner
Problem behavior begins shortly after owner
  leaves
May even occur during short absences
Pet shows exuberant greeting behavior

### GENERALIZED ANXIETY
Poorly socialized, nervous pet

### SIGNS OF ANXIETY
Hypervigilance, scanning
Increased motor activity (restlessness, pacing, circling)
Vocalization/whining
Displacement behaviors: out-of-context grooming and
  scratching, yawning, lip licking, whining and barking,
  destructive, digging
Changes in social soliciting behavior: increase or
  decrease in attention seeking
Hiding, escape attempts

Physiologic signs (trembling, dilated pupils, ptyalism, piloerection, ↑ respiratory rate, ↑ heart rate, urination, defecation, vomiting, anal sac expression)
Decreased appetite

## Ascites

See **Abdominal Effusions and Ascites**.

## Ataxia and Incoordination

### Forebrain Disease

Typically, mild ataxia and other neurologic signs predominate
Generalized disease: generalized ataxia
Unilateral disease: contralateral conscious proprioceptive deficits, mild gait disturbance
Postictal paraparesis: transient in nature
Paraparesis may be a side effect of anticonvulsant therapy (especially potassium bromide)

### Brain Stem

Hemiparesis or tetraparesis
- Lesions severe enough to cause paralysis usually result in respiratory arrest
Vestibular nuclei may be affected, causing vestibular ataxia, head tilt, and nystagmus
- Distinguish central vestibular disease from peripheral vestibular disease by presence of ipsilateral conscious proprioceptive deficits

### Peripheral Vestibular Disease

Generalized ataxia accompanied by head tilt, rotary or horizontal nystagmus, positional strabismus, and oculovestibular eye movements
Conscious proprioceptive deficits absent

### Cerebellum

Lesions cause dysmetria, usually hypermetria
Broad-based stance
Intention tremor
Unilateral lesions cause ipsilateral signs

### Cervical Spinal Cord

May cause forelimb monoparesis (lesions affecting spinal segments C6–T2), hemiparesis, tetraparesis; may progress to paralysis

## Thoracic (T3–L3) Spinal Cord

Mild to marked rear limb ataxia, paraparesis, paraplegia, monoparesis, or monoplegia

Rear limb reflexes exaggerated

Reduced to absent panniculus reflex caudal to lesion

## Lumbosacral (L4–S2) Spinal Cord

Mild to marked rear limb ataxia, paraparesis, paraplegia, monoplegia

Reduced to absent rear limb reflexes

May see bladder and anal sphincter hypotonia

## Peripheral Nerve

Mild to marked ataxia, paresis, paralysis of one or more limbs

Degenerative, inflammatory, toxic, traumatic neuropathies

Hyporeflexia usually seen

Paresis or paralysis of muscle or muscles innervated by affected nerve

## Back pain

Intervertebral disc disease
Neoplasia
  • Primary or metastatic
  • Multiple myeloma
Discospondylitis
Vertebral fracture/luxation
Ischemic myelopathy
Acute noncompressive nucleus pulposus extrusion
Meningitis/meningomyelitis
Orthopedic spinal pain
  • Spondylosis deformans
  • Articular facet degenerative joint disease
  • Psoas muscle injury
Nonspinal pain
  • Acute thromboembolism (cats)
  • Abdominal pain mimicking spinal pain
  • Kidney pain
  • Polyarthritis (multiple joint pain)
  • Polymyopathy (diffuse muscle disease)

## Blindness

### Corneal Lesions

Edema (trauma, glaucoma, immune-mediated keratitis such
as keratouveitis caused by canine adenovirus-1, endothe-
lial dystrophy, neurotrophic keratitis)
Keratoconjunctivitis sicca
Exposure keratitis
Superficial keratitis (pannus)
Corneal melanosis (entropion, ectropion, lagophthalmos,
facial nerve paralysis)
Cellular infiltrate (bacterial, viral, fungal)
Dystrophies (lipid, genetic)
Fibrosis (scar)

### Aqueous Humor Lesions

Fibrin (anterior uveitis: many causes)
Hypopyon (immune-mediated, neoplastic [lymphosar-
coma], infectious [blastomycosis, cryptococcus, histoplasmosis, coccidioidomycosis, toxoplasmosis, FIP,
prototheceosis, brucellosis, septicemia])
Hyphema (trauma, blood-clotting deficiencies, ehrlichiosis,
rickettsia, systemic hypertension, retinal detachment,
neoplasia)
Lipid (hyperlipidemia with concurrent anterior uveitis to
disrupt the blood–aqueous barrier)

### Lens Lesions

Cataracts (genetic, metabolic/diabetic, nutritional, traumatic, toxic, retinal degeneration, hypocalcemia, electric
shock, chronic uveitis, lens luxation)

### Vitreous Humor Lesions

Hemorrhage (trauma, systemic hypertension, clotting deficiency, neoplasia, retinal detachment)
Hyalitis (numerous infectious diseases such as FIP, penetrating injury causing cellular infiltrate)

### Retinal Lesions

Glaucoma
Sudden acquired retinal degeneration syndrome (SARDS)
Progressive retinal atrophy
Central progressive retinal atrophy
Toxicity (fluoroquinolone administration in cats)
Systemic hypertension

Retinal detachment
- Exudative/transudative (systemic hypertension, mycoses, rickettsial, toxoplasmosis, viral, bacterial, fungal)
- Neoplasia
- Retinal dysplasia
- Hereditary/congenital (e.g., Collie eye anomaly)

## Failure to Transmit Visual Message

Viral infections (canine distemper, FIP)
Systemic and ocular mycoses (blastomycosis, cryptococcosis, histoplasmosis, coccidioidomycosis)
Neoplasia
Traumatic avulsion of optic nerve (traumatic proptosis)
Granulomatous meningoencephalitis
Hydrocephalus
Optic nerve hypoplasia
Coloboma
Immune-mediated optic neuritis

## Failure to Interpret Visual Message

Canine distemper virus
FIP
Granulomatous meningoencephalitis
Systemic mycoses
Trauma
Heat stroke
Hypoxia
Hydrocephalus
Hepatoencephalopathy
Neoplasia
Storage diseases
Postictal
Meningitis

## Bradycardia, Sinus

Normal variation (fit animal)
Hypothyroidism
Hypothermia
Drugs (tranquilizers, anesthetics, β-blockers, calcium entry blockers, digitalis)
Increased intracranial pressure
Brain stem lesion
Severe metabolic disease (e.g., uremia)
Ocular pressure
Carotid sinus pressure
High vagal tone

Cardiac arrest (before and after)
Sinus node disease
Airway obstruction (causing high vagal tone)

## Cachexia and Muscle Wasting (Sarcopenia)

### Cachexia

Certain chronic disease processes stimulate the release
of cytokines that suppress appetite and stimulate
hypercatabolism
Cardiac disease
End-stage renal disease
Chronic infection
Chronic fever
Chronic inflammation
Neoplasia

### Muscle Wasting (Sarcopenia)

#### ENDOCRINE DISEASE
Hyperadrenocorticism
Hyperthyroidism
Hyperparathyroidism

#### STARVATION
Underfeeding
Poor-quality feed
Competition for food
Dental disease
Lactation, pregnancy
Increased work
Extreme cold environment

#### IMPAIRED ABILITY TO USE OR RETAIN NUTRIENTS
Dysphagia, regurgitation, vomiting
Maldigestion
Malabsorption
Parasitism
Histoplasmosis
Exocrine pancreatic insufficiency
Diabetes mellitus
Protein-losing nephropathy or gastroenteropathy

#### INFLAMMATORY MYOPATHIES
Masticatory myositis
Dermatomyositis
Canine idiopathic polymyositis
Feline idiopathic polymyositis

### PROTOZOAL MYOSITIS
*Toxoplasma gondii*
*Neospora caninum*

### INHERITED MYOPATHIES
Muscular dystrophy
Hereditary Labrador Retriever myopathy

### NEUROLOGIC DISORDERS
Spinal and peripheral neuropathies
Disuse atrophy

## Collapse

## Differential Diagnosis of Collapse

### CARDIOVASCULAR
Congestive heart failure
Arrhythmia
Arterial thromboembolism
Pulmonary hypertension
Cardiac tamponade
Ruptured splenic hemangiosarcoma

### RESPIRATORY
Laryngeal paralysis
Tracheal collapse
Asthma
Brachycephalic upper airway disease
Pulmonary edema
Pleural effusion
Pneumonia
Pharyngeal or laryngeal obstruction (mass, foreign body)
Lung lobe torsion

### METABOLIC/ENDOCRINE
Anemia
Hypoglycemia
Shock
Sepsis
Heat stroke
Hypoadrenocorticism
Anaphylaxis
Hypocalcemia
Hypokalemia

### BRAIN/CRANIAL NERVES
Canine geriatric vestibular syndrome

Feline idiopathic vestibular syndrome
Hemorrhage
Neoplasia
Intoxication
Infarct
Encephalitis
Hydrocephalus

### SPINAL CORD

Intervertebral disc disease
Trauma
Neoplasia
Discospondylitis
Hemorrhage
Fibrocartilaginous embolism
Meningitis/myelitis
Cervical spondylotic myelopathy (wobblers)

### PARTIAL SEIZURES

Idiopathic epilepsy
Brain disease

### NEUROMUSCULAR/MUSCULOSKELETAL

Tick paralysis
Polyradiculoneuritis
Botulism
Myasthenia gravis
Polyarthritis, polyneuropathy, polymyositis

### EXERCISE-INDUCED COLLAPSE

## Compulsive Behavior Disorders

### Compulsive Disorders in Dogs

#### LOCOMOTOR

Spinning or tail chasing
Stereotypic pacing/circling/jumping
Fixation; staring/barking/freezing/scratching
Chasing lights, reflections, shadows
Barking; intense/rhythmic/difficult to interrupt
Head bob/tremor/head shaking
Attacking food bowl, attacking inanimate objects

#### APPARENT HALLUCINATORY

Air biting or fly snapping
Staring, freezing, startled
Star-/skygazing

### SELF-INJURIOUS OR SELF-DIRECTED

Tail attacking, mutilation, growl/attack legs or rear
Face rubbing/scratching
Acral lick dermatitis, licking/chewing/barbering
Nail biting
Flank sucking
Checking rear

### ORAL

Sucking/licking
Pica, rock chewing
Polydipsia/polyphagia
Licking of objects/owners

## Compulsive Disorders in Cats

### LOCOMOTOR

Skin ripple/agitation/running, feline hyperesthesia
Circling
Freezing
Excessive/intense chasing of imaginary objects
Excessive vocalization/howling

### APPARENT HALLUCINATORY

Staring at shadows/walls
Startle
Avoiding imaginary objects

### SELF-INJURIOUS OR SELF-DIRECTED

Tail attacking, mutilation, growl/attack legs or rear
Face scratching/rubbing
Chewing/licking/barbering/overgrooming
Nail biting
Hyperesthesia

### ORAL

Wool sucking
Pica
Polydipsia/polyphagia
Licking of objects/owners

## Constipation

### Dietary Causes

Excessive fiber in dehydrated patient
Ingestion of hair, bones, indigestible materials

### Colonic Obstruction

Deviation of rectal canal: perineal hernia

Intraluminal or intramural disorders
- Tumor
- Granuloma
- Cicatrix
- Rectal foreign body
- Congenital stricture

Pseudocoprostasis
Perineal hernia
Extraluminal disorders
- Tumor
- Granuloma
- Abscess
- Healed pelvic fracture
- Prostatomegaly
- Prostatic or paraprostatic cyst
- Sublumbar lymphadenopathy

## Behavioral or Environmental Causes

Change in routine
Soiled or absent litter box
Refusal to defecate in house
Inactivity

## Drugs

Opiates
Anticholinergics
Sucralfate
Barium

## Refusal to Defecate

Pain in rectal or perineal area (perianal fistulas)
Inability to posture to defecate (orthopedic or neurologic problem)

## Colonic Weakness

### SYSTEMIC DISEASE

Hypercalcemia
Hypokalemia
Hypothyroidism
Chagas disease

### LOCALIZED NEUROMUSCULAR DISEASE

Spinal cord disease
Pelvic nerve damage
Dysautonomia
Chronic dilatation of colon/irreversible stretching of colonic musculature

## Miscellaneous Causes

Severe dehydration
Idiopathic megacolon (cats)

## Coughing

### Disorders of Upper Airway

#### INFLAMMATORY

Pharyngitis
Tonsillitis
Tracheobronchitis
Chronic bronchitis
Allergic bronchitis
Bronchiectasis
Collapsed trachea
*Oslerus osleri* infection

#### NEOPLASTIC

Mediastinal
Laryngeal
Tracheal

#### ALLERGIC

Bronchial asthma

#### OTHER

Bronchial compression: left atrial enlargement, hilar
  lymphadenopathy
Foreign body
Inhalation
Tracheal stenosis

### Disorders of Lower Respiratory Tract

#### INFLAMMATORY

*Pneumonia*
Bacterial
Viral: canine distemper virus
Fungal: blastomycosis, histoplasmosis,
  coccidioidomycosis
Protozoal: toxoplasmosis, pneumocystis pneumonia
Aspiration pneumonia

*Granuloma, Abscess*

#### PARASITIC DISEASE

Heartworm disease (*Dirofilaria immitis*)
Lungworm disease (*Aelurostrongylus abstrusus*—
  cat; *Paragonimus kellicotti*—dog, cat; *Capillaria*

*aerophila*—dog, cat; *Filaroides hirthi*—dog; *Crenosoma vulpis*—dog; *Angiostrongylus vasorum*—dog)

## NEOPLASIA
Primary or metastatic
Lymphoma

## CARDIOVASCULAR
Left-sided heart failure: pulmonary edema
Pulmonary thromboembolism

## NONCARDIOGENIC PULMONARY EDEMA

## ALLERGIC
Eosinophilic pneumonitis
Eosinophilic pulmonary granulomatosis
Pulmonary infiltrate with eosinophils (PIE)

## OTHER
Lung lobe torsion
Systemic bleeding disorder
Pleural effusion
Neoplasia of chest wall

## Cyanosis

### Central (Generalized) Cyanosis

#### CARDIAC
*Intracardiac*
Tetralogy of Fallot
Atrial or ventricular septal defect with pulmonic stenosis, tricuspid valve dysplasia, or pulmonary hypertension
Transposition complexes (double-outlet right ventricle, other)

*Extracardiac*
Pulmonary arteriovenous fistulas
Patent ductus arteriosus (reversed)

#### PULMONARY
*Hypoventilation*
Pleural effusion
Pneumothorax
Respiratory muscle failure (fatigue, neuromuscular disease)
Anesthetic overdose
Primary neurologic disease

*Obstruction*
Laryngeal paralysis

Foreign body in airway
Mass lesion of large airway (neoplasia, parasitic, inflammatory)
Low oxygen concentration of inspired air (high altitude, anesthetic complications)

*Ventilation–Perfusion Mismatch*
Pulmonary thromboembolism
Pulmonary infiltrate (edema, inflammation/ infection, neoplasia, acute respiratory distress syndrome, chronic obstructive pulmonary disease, fibrosis, pulmonary contusions/hemorrhage)

*Methemoglobinemia*

## Peripheral (Regional) Cyanosis

Central cyanosis (heart failure)
Decreased arterial supply
Peripheral vasoconstriction (hypothermia, shock)
Arterial thromboembolism
Low cardiac output
Obstruction of venous drainage
- Tourniquet or foreign object (e.g., rubber band)
- Venous thrombosis
- Right-sided heart failure

## Differential Cyanosis

Cyanosis of the caudal but not cranial half of the body; associated with Eisenmenger syndrome

## Deafness

## Congenital Sensorineural Deafness

### INHERITED

Many breeds of dogs
- Dalmatians
- Merle or dapple coat patterns in Collies, Shetland Sheepdogs, Great Danes, Dachshunds
- Piebald pattern in Dalmatians, Bull Terriers, Great Pyrenees, Sealyham Terriers, Greyhounds, Bulldogs, and Beagles
- Many other dog breeds affected (Rhodesian Ridgeback and Doberman Pinscher)
White cats with blue irides and white coloration in some breeds of dogs

## Congenital Acquired Sensorineural Deafness

In utero exposure to bacteria, ototoxic drugs, low oxygen tensions, or trauma

## Acquired Late-Onset Conductive Deafness

Lack of transmission of sound through tympanic membrane and auditory ossicles
Otitis externa/media
Otic neoplasia
Polyps
Trauma-induced fluid accumulation in middle ear
Atresia of tympanum or ossicles
Fused ossicles
Stenosis of ear canal leading to accumulation of fluid in middle ear
Total ear canal ablation

## Acquired Late-Onset Sensorineural Deafness

Presbycusis (age-related hearing loss)
Ototoxicity
Chronic exposure to loud noise
Hypothyroidism
Trauma
Bony neoplasia

## Diarrhea, Acute

### Diet

Intolerance/allergy
Rapid dietary change
Bacterial food poisoning
Dietary indiscretion
Poor-quality food

### Parasites

Helminths
Protozoa (*Giardia, Trichomonas, Coccidia* spp.)

### Infections

Viral (parvovirus, coronavirus, feline leukemia virus [FeLV], feline immunodeficiency virus [FIV], canine distemper virus, rotavirus)
Bacterial (*Salmonella* spp., *Clostridium perfringens, Escherichia coli, Campylobacter jejuni, Yersinia enterocolitica*, other bacteria)
Rickettsial
• Salmon poisoning

### Other Causes

Hemorrhagic gastroenteritis
Stress

Intussusception
Irritable bowel syndrome
Toxins (chemicals, heavy metals, toxic plants, spoiled foods, garbage)
Drugs (antibiotics, cancer chemotherapeutic agents, anthelmintics, NSAIDs, digitalis, lactulose)
Pancreatitis
Hypoadrenocorticism
Pyometra
Peritonitis

## Diarrhea, Chronic

### Small Bowel Diarrhea

Food intolerance or allergy
Inflammatory bowel disease
GI lymphoma
Pancreatic exocrine insufficiency
Chronic parasitism (hookworm, *Giardia*)
Histoplasmosis
Intestinal lymphangiectasia
Partial obstruction
Pancreatic carcinoma
Gastrinoma
Liver disease (hepatocellular failure, cholestasis)
Endocrine disease (hypoadrenocorticism, hypothyroidism, hyperthyroidism)
Renal disease (uremia, nephrotic syndrome)
Chronic intussusception
Small intestinal bacterial overgrowth
Pythiosis

### Large Bowel Diarrhea

Food intolerance or allergy
Parasitism (whipworm, *Giardia, Trichomonas, Heterobilharzia*)
Clostridial colitis
Irritable bowel syndrome (fiber-responsive)
Histoplasmosis
Pythiosis
Inflammatory bowel disease
- Lymphocytic-plasmacytic colitis
- Eosinophilic colitis
- Chronic ulcerative colitis
- Histiocytic ulcerative colitis (Boxers)
Neoplasia (lymphoma, adenocarcinoma)
FeLV/FIV (infections secondary to these viruses)

## Dyschezia

See **Tenesmus and Dyschezia**

## Dysphagia

### Oral Lesions

Fractured bones or teeth
Periodontitis
Trauma (laceration, hematoma)
Feline resorptive lesions (caries)
Osteomyelitis
Retrobulbar abscess/inflammation
Temporal–masseter myositis
Stomatitis, glossitis, pharyngitis, gingivitis, tonsillitis, sialadenitis
- Immune-mediated disease
- Feline herpesvirus, calicivirus, leukemia virus, immunodeficiency virus
- Lingual foreign bodies or granulomas
- Tooth root abscess
- Uremia
- Caustic chemicals
Cleft palate
Lingual frenulum disorder
Cricopharyngeal achalasia/asynchrony

### Obstructive Lesion

Esophageal stricture/foreign object
Esophagitis
Electric cord burns
Neoplasia (malignant or benign)
Inflammatory (abscess, polyp, granuloma)
Lymphadenopathy
Eosinophilic granuloma
Foreign object (oral, pharyngeal, laryngeal)
Sialocele
Nasopharyngeal polyp

### Neuromuscular Disease

Myasthenia gravis
Acute polyradiculitis
Masticatory myositis
Tick paralysis
Botulism
Polymyositis
Temporomandibular joint disease

Rabies
Trigeminal nerve paralysis or neuritis
Neuropathies of cranial nerves V, VII, IX, X, or XII
Brain stem disease
Tetanus
Hypothyroidism

## Dyspnea

### Inspiratory Dyspnea

#### NASAL OBSTRUCTION

Rhinitis
- Viral: feline herpesvirus, feline calicivirus, canine distemper virus
- Bacterial
- Fungal: aspergillosis, cryptococcosis, penicilliosis, rhinosporidiosis

Neoplasia: adenocarcinoma, squamous cell carcinoma, fibrosarcoma, osteosarcoma, chondrosarcoma, lymphoma, transmissible venereal tumor
Stenotic nares
Nasal foreign body
Thick nasal discharge of any etiology

#### PHARYNGEAL OR LARYNGEAL DISEASE

Elongated soft palate, everted laryngeal saccules
Neoplasia/mass, abscess, granuloma, extraluminal mass
Nasopharyngeal polyp
Foreign body
Laryngeal paralysis, acute/obstructive laryngitis, laryngeal collapse, laryngeal trauma
Cricopharyngeal achalasia

#### EXTRATHORACIC TRACHEA

Collapsing trachea
Tracheal hypoplasia
Tracheal trauma/stricture, foreign body, neoplasia

### Expiratory or Mixed Dyspnea

#### INTRATHORACIC TRACHEA AND BRONCHI

Collapsing trachea or main-stem bronchus
Trauma, stricture, foreign body, neoplasia
Small airway disease
Feline asthma
Bronchitis
Smoke inhalation
Bronchopneumonia

## PULMONARY PARENCHYMAL DISEASE
Pneumonia (viral, bacterial, fungal, protozoal, aspiration)
Pulmonary edema
Pulmonary thromboembolism
Bronchial asthma
Chronic obstructive lung disease

## PARASITES/SEVERE INFESTATIONS/HEARTWORM, LUNGWORMS
Pulmonary fibrosis
Neoplasia

## PLEURAL SPACE DISEASE
Pleural effusion
Pneumothorax
Pleural space masses
Diaphragmatic hernia

## NONCARDIOPULMONARY DISEASE
Severe anemia
Hypovolemia
Acidosis
Hyperthermia
Neurologic disease

# Dysuria

See **Stranguria, Dysuria, and Pollakiuria**

# Ecchymoses

See **Petechiae and Ecchymoses**

# Edema

## Increased Hydrostatic Pressure

### IMPAIRED VENOUS RETURN
Congestive heart failure
Constrictive pericarditis
Ascites (cirrhosis)
Budd-Chiari syndrome
Venous obstruction or compression (thrombosis, external pressure, extremity inactivity)
Iatrogenic overhydration
Heartworm disease

### SMALL-CALIBER ARTERIOLAR DILATATION
Heat
Neurohumoral dysregulation

## Reduced Plasma Osmotic Pressure

### HYPOPROTEINEMIA
Cirrhosis (ascites)
Malnutrition
Protein-losing enteropathy
Protein-losing glomerulonephropathy (nephrotic syndrome)
Lymphangiectasia

## Lymphatic Obstruction

Various inflammatory causes
Neoplasia
Postsurgical
After radiation therapy

## Sodium Retention

Excessive dietary intake with renal disease
Renal hypoperfusion
Increased renin–angiotensin–aldosterone secretion

## Inflammation

Acute and chronic
Angiogenesis

## Increased Microvascular Permeability

Sepsis
Acute respiratory distress syndrome
Pancreatitis
Infection (fungal, bacterial, viral)
Envenomation
Burns
Myxedema

## Mixed Mechanisms

Noncardiogenic pulmonary edema (head trauma, seizures, electrocution, upper airway obstruction)
Anaphylaxis
Organ torsion

## Epistaxis

## Systemic Causes

Thrombocytopenia
- Decreased production of thrombocytes (infectious, myelophthisis secondary to neoplasia, drugs, immune-mediated phenomena)

- Increased destruction (immune-mediated, microangiopathy)
- Increased consumption (DIC, vasculitis, hemorrhage)

Thrombocytopathia

- Primary (von Willebrand disease)
- Secondary (uremia, ehrlichiosis, multiple myeloma, drugs such as NSAIDs)

Coagulation factor defects (e.g., hemophilia A and B)

Acquired coagulopathies (anticoagulant rodenticides, hepatic failure)

Increased capillary fragility (hypertension, hyperviscosity syndromes [multiple myeloma, ehrlichiosis, leishmaniasis], hyperlipidemia, thromboembolic disease)

Polycythemia

Systemic hypertension

## Local Causes

Neoplasia (nasal adenocarcinoma, lymphoma, benign polyps)

Foreign body

Bacterial infection (usually secondary; rarely, *Bordetella*, *Pasteurella*, or *Mycoplasma* can be primary cause of epistaxis)

Fungal rhinitis (*Aspergillus*, *Cryptococcus* spp.)

Dental disease with oronasal fistulation

Trauma

Nasal parasites: *Pneumonyssus caninum* (nasal mite), *Eucoleus boehmi* (formerly *Capillaria* spp.), *Cuterebra* spp.

Eosinophilic and lymphoplasmacytic rhinitis (uncommon)

Arteriovenous malformations

## Erosions and Ulcers of Skin and Mucous Membranes

### Canine Diseases

#### INFECTIOUS

Bacterial pyoderma

Surface: acute moist dermatitis (pyotraumatic dermatitis), intertrigo

Deep: folliculitis/furunculosis (including pyotraumatic folliculitis), oral bacterial infections

#### FUNGAL

Yeast infections (*Malassezia pachydermatis*, *Candida* spp.), systemic/subcutaneous

#### PARASITIC

Demodicosis

## METABOLIC
Calcinosis cutis (hyperadrenocorticism)
Uremia/renal failure
Necrolytic migratory erythema/metabolic epidermal
 necrosis

## NEOPLASTIC
Epitheliotropic lymphoma
Squamous cell carcinoma

## PHYSICAL/CHEMICAL
Drug reactions
Solar injury
Thermal injury (freeze, burn)
Urine scald

## IMMUNE-MEDIATED/AUTOIMMUNE
DLE, vesicular cutaneous erythematosus
Pemphigus group
Uveodermatologic syndrome
Miscellaneous autoimmune subepidermal vesiculobullous diseases: bullous pemphigoid, epidermolysis
 bullosa acquisita, linear immunoglobulin IgA bullous
 disease, mucocutaneous pemphigoid, bullous systemic
 lupus type 1

## MISCELLANEOUS
Arthropod bites
Dermatomyositis
Dystrophic epidermolysis bullosa
Idiopathic ulceration of Collies
Junctional epidermolysis bullosa
Toxic epidermal necrolysis/erythema multiforme
- Junctional epidermolysis bullosa
- Acral mutilation syndrome (French Spaniels, German
  and English Pointers)
- Cutaneous asthenia (Ehler-Danlos syndrome)

## Feline Diseases

## INFECTIOUS
Viral: calicivirus and herpesvirus
Bacterial: atypical mycobacteriosis
Fungal: subcutaneous (e.g., sporotrichosis) and systemic
 mycoses (e.g., cryptococcosis)

## METABOLIC
Uremia/renal disease

## NEOPLASTIC
Fibrosarcoma

Lymphoma

Squamous cell carcinoma

## PHYSICAL/CHEMICAL

Drug reactions

Thermal

## IMMUNE-MEDIATED/AUTOIMMUNE

Bullous pemphigoid

Pemphigus foliaceous

Toxic epidermal necrolysis/erythema multiforme

## MISCELLANEOUS/IDIOPATHIC

Arthropod bites

Dystrophic epidermolysis bullosa

Eosinophilic plaque

Idiopathic ulceration of dorsal neck

Indolent ulcer

Junctional epidermolysis bullosa

- Skin fragility syndrome
- Cutaneous asthenia (Ehler-Danlos syndrome)

# Failure to Grow/Failure to Thrive

## Small Stature and Poor Body Condition

Dietary insufficiency

Underfeeding

Poor-quality diet

GI disease

- Parasitism
- Inflammatory bowel disease
- Food intolerance/allergy
- Obstruction (foreign body, intussusception)
- Histoplasmosis

Hepatic dysfunction

- Portovascular anomaly
- Hepatitis
- Glycogen storage disease

Cardiac disorder

- Congenital anomaly
- Endocarditis

Pulmonary disease

Esophageal disease

- Megaesophagus
- Vascular ring anomaly (persistent right aortic arch)

Exocrine pancreatic insufficiency

Renal disease

Renal failure (congenital or acquired)

- Glomerular disease
- Pyelonephritis

Inflammatory disease

Glycogen storage disease

Hormonal disease

- Diabetes mellitus
- Hypoadrenocorticism
- Diabetes insipidus
- Juvenile hyperparathyroidism

## Small Stature and Good Body Condition

Chondrodystrophy

Hormonal disease

- Congenital hypothyroidism
- Congenital hyposomatotropism (pituitary dwarfism)
- Hyperadrenocorticism

## Fever of Unknown Origin

### Infection

#### BACTERIAL

Abscessation (inapparent subcutaneous, stump pyometra, liver, pancreas, tooth root, retrobulbar)

Pyelonephritis

Discospondylitis

Osteomyelitis

Pneumonia

Prostatitis

Peritonitis

Pyothorax

Closed pyometra

Splenic abscess

Septic arthritis

Sepsis

Cholangiohepatitis (cat)

Bartonellosis

*Mycoplasma haemofelis* (formerly *Hemobartonella felis*)

Borreliosis

Brucellosis

Leptospirosis

Mycobacteriosis L-form bacteria (cat)

Mycoplasmosis

Salmonellosis

Tularemia

Bacterial endocarditis

Plague

Tuberculosis

#### FUNGAL
Blastomycosis
Histoplasmosis
Coccidioidomycosis
Cryptococcosis
Systemic aspergillosis

#### VIRAL
Canine distemper
Canine influenza
FIV
FeLV
FIP *(Coronavirus)*
Feline calicivirus, feline herpesvirus 1

#### RICKETTSIAL
Rocky Mountain spotted fever
Ehrlichiosis
Anaplasmosis
Salmon poisoning

#### PROTOZOAL
Toxoplasmosis
Babesiosis
Hepatozoonosis
Cytauxzoonosis
Trypanosomiasis (Chagas disease)
Leishmaniasis
Neosporosis

## Neoplasia

Lymphoma
Multiple myeloma
Leukemia
Histiocytic sarcoma
Necrotic solid tumors

## Immune-Mediated

Polyarthritis
Vasculitis
Meningitis
SLE
Pemphigus
Rheumatoid arthritis
Immune-mediated hemolytic anemia
Immune-mediated thrombocytopenia
Meningoencephalitis (granulomatous, necrotizing)
Steroid-responsive fever
Steroid-responsive neutropenia

## Inflammatory

- Hypertrophic osteodystrophy
- Juvenile cellulitis
- Pancreatitis
- Panniculitis
- Panosteitis
- Pansteatitis

## Other

Hyperthyroidism
Tissue damage
Pharmacologic agents
- Tetracycline
- Penicillins
- Sulfas

Metabolic bone disease
Portosystemic shunt
Hypothalamic disease
Shar-Pei fever
Idiopathic

## Flatulence

Dietary intolerance (high-fiber, high-protein, or high-fat foods; high-sulfur diets; spoiled food; food change)
Maldigestion
- Exocrine pancreatic insufficiency
- Lactose intolerance

Malabsorption
Motility disorders (disrupt passage of gas)
Aerophagia (brachycephalic breeds)
Behavior (aerophagia associated with competitive eating habits)
Various GI disorders

## Gagging

### Nutritional

Food texture
Food size

### Infectious

Viral encephalitis (rabies, pseudorabies)
Fungal (focal, systemic)
Bacterial encephalitis

## Toxic

Chemical (caustic chemicals, smoke)
Botulism

## Developmental

Cleft palate
Hydrocephalus
Achalasia

## Degenerative

Laryngeal paralysis
Muscular dystrophy
Myasthenia gravis
Neuropathy of cranial nerves V, VII, IX, or XII

## Mechanical

Foreign body
Styloid disarticulation

## Metabolic

Uremia
Hypocalcemia

## Neoplasia

Tonsils, pharynx, epiglottis, glottis, inner ear, nasal, CNS

## Trauma

Tracheal rupture
Pharyngeal hematoma
Medulla or pons ischemia or edema

## Allergic or Immune-Mediated

Rhinitis
Pharyngitis
Laryngitis
Asthma
Granuloma complex
Idiopathic glossopharyngitis

## Genital Dermatoses

### Lesions of the Prepuce/Sheath

Bacterial folliculitis/furunculosis
Allergic dermatitis affecting the abdomen with hyperpigmentation/lichenification/hypertrophy of the sheath
Localized demodicosis

Vasculitis

Autoimmune skin diseases

Linear dermatosis of the prepuce (estrogen-secreting tumor)

Linear epidermal nevus

Vascular nevus

Various neoplasms (Stricker sarcoma, hemangiosarcoma, mast cell tumor)

## Lesions of the Scrotum

Contact dermatitis (most common scrotal skin disease)

Frostbite, solar erythema, trauma

Intertrigo

*Malassezia* dermatitis

Prototheosis

Babesiosis

Cuterebriasis

Brucellosis

Infection with *Erysipelothrix rhusiopathiae*

Rocky Mountain spotted fever

Superficial necrolytic dermatitis

Autoimmune diseases (bullous diseases, lupus)

Erythema multiforme

Fixed pigmented erythema

Cutaneous histiocytosis

Vascular hamartoma

Neoplasms (squamous cell carcinoma, apocrine adenocarcinoma, myxoma and fibrosarcoma, hemangioma, recurrent cystic hemangioma and hemangiosarcoma, plasmocytoma, lymphoma, histiocytoma, benign fibrous histiocytoma, mast cell tumor, melanoma)

## Lesions of the Female Genitalia

Intertrigo

Allergic dermatitis affecting the abdomen with hyperpigmentation/lichenification/hypertrophy of the vulva

*Malassezia* dermatitis

Demodicosis

Bacterial furunculosis

Contact dermatitis

Autoimmune diseases (lupus, bullous diseases)

Endocrine disorders (especially hyperestrogenism)

Neoplasms

# Halitosis

## Oral Disease

Periodontal disease (gingivitis, periodontitis, abscessation)

Calculus
Food traps (periodontal pockets, exposed tooth roots, oral ulcers)
Neoplasia (melanoma, fibrosarcoma, squamous cell carcinoma)
Foreign body
Trauma/fracture
Electric cord injury
Pharyngitis
Stomatitis/glossitis
Congenital and acquired palate defects
Oronasal fistula

## Metabolic Disease

Renal failure (uremia)
Diabetic ketoacidosis

## Gastrointestinal Disease

Megaesophagus
Inflammatory bowel disease
Exocrine pancreatic insufficiency
Neoplasia
Constipation

## Respiratory Disease

Rhinitis/sinusitis
Neoplasia
Pneumonia or pulmonary abscess

## Dermatologic Disease

Lip fold pyoderma
Eosinophilic granuloma
Ulcerative mucocutaneous pyoderma
Pemphigus complex
Bullous pemphigoid
Lupus erythematosus
Drug eruption
Cutaneous lymphoma
Exposure to dimethyl sulfoxide (DMSO)

## Dietary

Aromatic foods (onions, garlic)
Fetid food (carrion)
Coprophagy

## Grooming Behavior

Anal sacculitis
Vaginitis/balanoposthitis
Lower urinary tract infections
Hair retained in periodontal pockets

## Head Tilt

### Peripheral Vestibular Disease

Otitis media/interna
Feline idiopathic vestibular disease
Geriatric canine vestibular disease
Feline nasopharyngeal polyps
Middle ear tumor
- Ceruminous gland adenocarcinoma
- Squamous cell carcinoma

Trauma
Aminoglycoside ototoxicity
Hypothyroidism (possibly)
Congenital (German Shepherd, Doberman Pinscher,
    English Cocker Spaniel, Siamese and Burmese cats)

### Central Vestibular Disease

Trauma/hemorrhage
Infectious inflammatory disease
- Rocky Mountain spotted fever
- FIP
- Bacterial
- Protozoal
- Mycotic
- Rickettsial
- Others

Granulomatous meningoencephalitis
Neoplasia (meningioma, choroid plexus tumors)
Vascular infarct
Thiamine deficiency
Metronidazole toxicity
Viral (canine distemper virus, FIP)
Toxic (lead, hexachlorophene)
Degenerative diseases (storage diseases, neuronopathies,
    demyelinating diseases)
Hydrocephalus

## Hematemesis

### Alimentary Tract Lesion

#### GASTRITIS

Acute gastritis (common cause)
Hemorrhagic gastroenteritis
Chronic gastritis
*Helicobacter*-associated disease

**FOREIGN BODY**

**HEAVY METAL INTOXICATION**
Arsenic, lead, zinc

**GASTROINTESTINAL TRACT ULCERATION/EROSION**
*Iatrogenic*
NSAIDs
Corticosteroids
NSAIDs used in combination with corticosteroids

## Infiltrative Disease

Neoplasia
Inflammatory bowel disease
Pythiosis (young dogs, southeastern United States)
Stress ulceration
- Hypovolemic shock
- Septic shock
- After gastric dilatation/volvulus
- Neurogenic shock
Burns
Multiple trauma
Hyperacidity
- Mast cell tumor
- Gastrinoma (rare)
Other causes
- Hepatic disease
- Renal disease
- Hypoadrenocorticism
- Inflammatory disease

**ESOPHAGEAL DISEASE (UNCOMMON)**
Tumor
Severe esophagitis
Trauma

**BLEEDING ORAL LESION**

**GALLBLADDER DISEASE (RARE)**

## Coagulopathy

Thrombocytopenia/platelet dysfunction
Clotting factor deficiency
DIC
Anticoagulant rodenticide

## Extraalimentary Tract Lesion

Respiratory tract lesion
Lung lobe torsion

Pulmonary tumor
Posterior nares lesion

## Hematochezia

### Anal Disease

Perianal fistulas
Anal sacculitis or abscess
Stricture
Neoplasia (perianal adenoma, anal sac adenocarcinoma)
Anal trauma
Perineal hernia
Foreign body

### Rectal and Colonic Disease

Hemorrhagic gastroenteritis
Proctitis
Colitis
* Idiopathic
* Dietary allergy
* Inflammatory bowel disease
* Stress
* Infectious (*Campylobacter* spp., *Clostridium perfringens*)
* Histoplasmosis
* Pythiosis
* Food allergy
* Trichomoniasis (cat)
Parvovirus
Parasites
* Whipworms
* Hookworms
* Coccidia
Neoplasia
* Rectal polyp
* Adenocarcinoma
* Lymphoma
* Leiomyoma or leiomyosarcoma
Prolapsed rectum
Mucosal trauma
* Foreign body or foreign material
* Pelvic fractures
* Iatrogenic (thermometers, enemas, fecal loops, rectal palpation)
Iliocecal intussusceptions

## Hematuria

### Renal or Lower Urinary Tract Disease

Inflammation/infection
Urolithiasis
Obstruction
Trauma (catheter collection, cystocentesis, renal biopsy,
 blunt trauma)
Neoplasia
Bleeding disorder (anticoagulant intoxication, DIC,
 thrombocytopenia)
Heat stroke
Renal infarct
Granulomatous urethritis
Feline lower urinary tract disease (FLUTD)
Parasitism (*Dioctophyma renale, Capillaria plica*)
Drug-induced (cyclophosphamide)
Renal pelvic hematoma
Vascular malformation
Idiopathic renal hematuria
Renal telangiectasia of Welsh Corgis
Renal hematuria of Weimaraners
Pseudohematuria (myoglobin, hemoglobin, drugs, dyes)

### Extraurinary Disease

Prostatic disease (infection, tumor, cyst, abscess)
Uterine disease (pyometra, proestrus, tumor, subinvolution
 of placental sites)
Vaginal (trauma, neoplasia)
Estrus
Preputial/penile (trauma, neoplasia)

## Hemoptysis

### Cardiovascular

Heartworm disease
Cardiogenic pulmonary edema
Arteriovenous fistula
Bacterial endocarditis

### Pulmonary

Thromboembolism (secondary to neoplasia, endocrine,
 cardiac, metabolic disease)
Bacterial pneumonia

Pulmonary abscess
Nocardiosis
*Bordetella bronchiseptica* infection
Chronic bronchitis/bronchiectasis
Fungal pneumonia (blastomycosis, coccidiomycosis,
   histoplasmosis)
Neoplasia (hemangiosarcoma, primary adenocarcinoma,
   undifferentiated carcinoma, squamous cell carcinoma,
   chondrosarcoma, metastatic or primary tracheal tumors)
Lung lobe torsion
Parasites (*Paragonimus kellicotti, Capillaria aerophila,
   Aelurostrongylus abstrusus*)
Pulmonary infiltrate with eosinophils
Systemic bleeding disorder
• Primary (quantitative or qualitative platelet defects)
• Secondary (factor deficiencies, anticoagulant rodenticide
   toxicity, DIC)
Trauma (pulmonary contusion, tracheal rupture, inhaled
   foreign body)
Iatrogenic (endotracheal intubation, complication of lung
   biopsy/aspirate, transtracheal wash, bronchoscopy)

## Hemorrhage, Prolonged

See **Part Two**, Section V: **Differential Diagnosis for Thrombocytopenia, Platelet Dysfunction, and Coagulopathies, Inherited and Acquired**

## Horner Syndrome

2.5% phenylephrine eye drops applied

### No Pupillary Dilation (Assume Preganglionic Lesion)

First order (central)
Intracranial disease (neoplasia, trauma, infarct)
First cervical to third thoracic (C1–T3) spinal myelopathy
   (intervertebral disc disease, neoplasia, fibrocartilaginous
   embolism, trauma)
Second order (preganglionic)
Spinal cord lesion T1–T3 (trauma, neoplasia, fibrocartilagi-
   nous embolism)
Thoracic disease (cranial mediastinal mass, thoracic spinal
   nerve root tumor)
Brachial plexus avulsion
Cervical soft tissue neoplasia, trauma
Skull base tumor
Jugular furrow disease

## Pupillary Dilation (Assume Postganglionic Lesion)

Third order (postganglionic)
  FeLV, FIV
  Otitis media/interna
  Otic mass
  Retrobulbar injury, neoplasia
  Idiopathic

## Hyperemia

### Differential Diagnosis of Hyperemia

#### REGIONAL HYPEREMIA
  Allergen exposure (contact, insect/mite bite)
  External constriction (rubber band, collar, identification band, tight bandage)
  Internal obstruction

#### GENERALIZED HYPEREMIA
  Hyperthermia-induced (infectious, inflammatory, immune-mediated, neurogenic, environmental, toxic)
  Anaphylaxis/drug reaction
  Mast cell tumor
  Contact dermatitis
  Carbon monoxide intoxication
  Pheochromocytoma
  Decreased venous return (cardiac, hepatic, venous occlusion)
  Hyperdynamic phase of shock
  Drugs and toxins (alpha-adrenergic receptor blocker, alcohol, cyanide, acepromazine)
  Erythrocytosis
  Hemoglobinemia

## Hyperpigmentation

Increased melanin in the epidermis

### Hereditary Hyperpigmentation

Lentigines—darkly pigmented macules that develop on the ventral abdomen of healthy adult dogs and on the lips, nose, gingiva, and eyelids of orange cats. No adverse health effects.

Canine acanthosis nigricans—bilateral hyperpigmentation and lichenification of axillary skin. Primary, hereditary form seen in Dachshunds beginning before age 1. When seen in older Dachshunds or other breeds, it is likely a postinflammatory form seen with friction, intertrigo, allergies, or endocrine disease.

Acromelanism—dark areas on the points of Siamese, Himalayan-Persian, Balinese, and Burmese cats. Result of a temperature-dependent enzyme controlling melanin production in hair bulbs.

## Acquired Hyperpigmentation

Postinflammatory—Mediators of inflammation (e.g., leukotrienes, thromboxanes) stimulate melanocytes to increase melanin production, which downregulates inflammation by scavenging free radicles. Examples of inflammatory conditions that lead to increased melanin production include allergies, *Malassezia* dermatitis, bacterial pyoderma, dermatophytosis, demodicosis, scabies, and actinic and intertrigo dermatitis. Inflammation affecting hair follicles may lead to melanotrichia (e.g., sebaceous adenitis, panniculitis, vaccine reactions).

Endocrine—hyperadrenocorticism, hypoadrenocorticism, hypothyroidism, hyperestrogenism, and other sex hormone imbalances may result in diffuse hyperpigmentation.

Papillomavirus-associated—Pugs may be at risk for development of papillomavirus-associated, slightly raised, scaly, hyperpigmented macules and plaques in their groin region, abdomen, ventral thorax, and neck. Similar lesions are described in Miniature Schnauzers, American Staffordshire Terriers, and Pomeranians. May transform to squamous cell carcinoma.

Pigmented tumors—apocrine cysts are bluish, cutaneous hemangiomas and hemangiosarcomas appear red, dark purple, or bluish-black. Melanomas, melanocytomas, and basal cell tumors are frequently black. Squamous cell carcinomas, trichoblastomas, and fibromas also may be dark brown to black.

## Hyperthermia

### Fever

Exogenous pyrogens (infectious agents and their products, inflammation or necrosis of tissue, immune complexes, pharmacologic agents, bile acids)

Endogenous pyrogens (fever-producing cytokines)

### Heat Stroke

High ambient temperatures

Exercise
Poor ventilation
Brachycephalic conformation
Obesity

## Exercise Hyperthermia

Sustained exercise
Seizure disorders (especially prolonged or cluster seizures)
Hypocalcemic tetany (eclampsia)
Tremorgenic toxins (metaldehyde, mycotoxins, permethrin)

## Pathologic Etiologies

Lesions in or around anterior hypothalamus
Hypermetabolic disorders
Hyperthyroidism
Pheochromocytoma
Malignant hyperthermia
Halothane
Succinylcholine
Phenothiazines

## Hypopigmentation

Due to melanocyte destruction, dysfunction, or abnormal
distribution of melanosomes

## Hereditary Hypopigmentation

Albinism—hereditary absence of pigment
Piebaldism—presence of white spots where melanocytes are
absent
Waardenburg-Klein syndrome—affected animals have
absence of melanocytes in areas of skin and hair, blue
or heterochromatic eyes, and are also deaf. Reported
in cats, Bull Terriers, Sealyham Terriers, Collies, and
Dalmatians.
Canine cyclic hematopoiesis—lethal autosomal-recessive
disease of Collies. Gray coat, light-colored nose, cyclic
episodes of neutropenia every 12–14 days resulting in
sepsis and amyloidosis.
Chédiak-Higashi syndrome—rare autosomal-recessive
disease of blue smoke Persian cats. Partial oculocutane-
ous albinism with abnormal function of granulocytes
and platelets resulting in hemorrhage, recurrent infections, and death at a young age.
Graying—age-associated reduction of melanocyte
replication

Vitiligo—macular leukoderma and leukotrichia of nose, ears, buccal mucosa, and facial skin. Antimelanocyte antibodies found in serum of some affected dogs. Seen most commonly in Siamese cats, Belgian Tervuren, German Shepherd, Collie, Rottweiler, Doberman Pinscher, Giant Schnauzer.

Nasal hypopigmentation—season-associated lightening of nasal planum during winter months; most common in Siberian Husky, Golden Retriever, Labrador Retriever, and Bernese Mountain Dog. Seen also in many other breeds.

Mucocutaneous hypopigmentation—leukoderma of the nasal planum, lips, eyelids, tongue, and oral cavity. Many breeds of dogs, but more common in Australian Shepherds, Siberian Huskies, Golden Retrievers, and Labrador Retrievers. Congenital condition in Rottweilers and Doberman Pinschers.

Tyrosinase deficiency—rare condition in Chow Chows. Puppies show dramatic color change, bluish-black tongue turns pink, hair shafts turn white. Melanin reappears spontaneously in 2–4 months.

## Acquired Hypopigmentation

Postinflammatory—DLE is the most common cause of postinflammatory nasal depigmentation. Also pemphigus complex, SLE, uveodermatologic syndrome, bullous pemphigoid, mucocutaneous pyoderma, drug eruption, and contact dermatitis. Infectious causes include leishmaniasis, blastomycosis, sporotrichosis, and bacterial folliculitis.

Drug related—ketoconazole, procainamide, and vitamin E may cause diffuse coat lightening.

Nutritional/metabolic—deficiencies of zinc, pyridoxine, pantothenic acid, and lysine are associated with graying of hair. Dark hairs may become reddish in color with copper deficiency, hypothyroidism, hyperadrenocorticism, hyperestrogenism, hyperprogesteronism, chlorine exposure, and chronic exposure to ultraviolet light.

Neoplasia associated—nasal depigmentation, leukoderma, and leukotrichia; sometimes seen with epitheliotropic T-cell lymphoma, basal cell tumors, mammary adenocarcinoma, and gastric carcinomas.

Idiopathic—leukotrichia and patchy hypopigmentation reported as idiopathic in Labrador Retrievers and black Newfoundlands. Siamese cats may be affected with periocular leukotrichia, which may be associated with upper respiratory tract infections, pregnancy, dietary deficiencies, or systemic illness.

## Hyphema

### Causes of Hyphema

#### GENETIC/BREED PREDISPOSITION

- Hereditary coagulopathies
- Breeds predisposed to retinal detachment
  Retinal dysplasia: presumed autosomal-recessive trait,
    (English Springer Spaniel, Bedlington Terrier, American
    Cocker Spaniel, Miniature Schnauzer); incomplete
    dominant inheritance in breeds with associated skeletal
    deformities (Labrador Retriever, Samoyed)
  Multifocal retinopathy: autosomal recessive in Coton de
    Tulear, Great Pyrenees, Australian Shepherd
  Collie eye anomaly (Collies, Shetland Sheepdog, Border
    Collie, Australian Shepherd)
  Shih Tzus are predisposed to vitreous degeneration and
    rhegmatogenous (retina is torn) retinal detachments
- Persistent hyperplastic primary vitreous in Doberman
  Pinschers

#### STIMULI FOR INTRAOCULAR NEOVASCULARIZATION

Retinal detachments
Intraocular neoplasia
Glaucoma
Uveitis

#### PREDISPOSITION TO OCULAR TRAUMA

Blind animals
Hunting dogs
Exophthalmic animals
Puppies exposed to cats

#### SYSTEMIC DISEASES THAT CAUSE VASCULOPATHY AND/OR BLEEDING DISORDERS

Systemic hypertension
Lymphoma
Hyperviscosity syndromes (multiple myeloma, polycy-
  themia vera)
Infectious disease (FeLV, FIP, rickettsial diseases)
Immune-mediated thrombocytopenia or anemia
Anticoagulation rodenticide intoxication
Severe hepatic disease

## Hypothermia

### Predisposing Factors

Anesthesia
Low ambient temperature

Neonate
Small size
Elderly
Sick
Debilitated
Near drowning
Enema

## Systemic Disease

Cardiac disease
Hypothyroidism
Sepsis
Chronic kidney disease
Hypoadrenocorticism
Malnourished
Hypoglycemia
Neurologic disease (head trauma, neoplasia, cerebral vascular disease)

# Icterus (Jaundice)

## Hemolysis

Autoimmune hemolytic anemia
Hemolytic anemia secondary to drugs, neoplasia
Infectious (*Ehrlichia canis, Babesia canis, Babesia felis, Mycoplasma hemocanis, Mycoplasma hemofelis, Cytauxzoon felis*, heartworm disease, FeLV)
Toxic (onions, lead, copper, methylene blue, benzocaine, propylene glycol, acetaminophen [cats], phenazopyridine)
Fragmentation (DIC, hemangiosarcoma, vena cava syndrome)
Erythrocyte membrane or enzyme defects (pyruvate kinase deficiency [Beagle, Basenji], phosphofructokinase deficiency [English Springer Spaniel], stomatocytosis of chondrodysplastic [Malamutes])
Congenital porphyria
Snake, brown recluse spider, and bee venoms

## Hepatobiliary Disease

Cholangiohepatitis
Chronic inflammatory hepatic disease
Cirrhosis
Diffuse neoplasia
Infection (leptospirosis, histoplasmosis, infectious canine hepatitis, FIP, sepsis)
Copper toxicity

Toxic hepatopathy (anticonvulsants, mebendazole, oxi-
bendazole, diethylcarbamazine, inhalation anesthetics,
thiacetarsamide, acetaminophen, trimethoprim-sulfa,
sago palm, blue-green algae)
Hepatic lipidosis
FIP
Parasitic
Idiosyncratic drug reaction

## Posthepatic Biliary Obstruction

Pancreatitis
Enteritis/cholecystitis
Trauma
Neoplasia
Calculus
Stricture
Mucocele
Ruptured bile duct or gallbladder

## Inappropriate Elimination

### Dogs

#### MEDICAL CAUSES

*Fecal House Soiling*

Increased volume of feces (maldigestion, malabsorp-
tion, high-fiber diets)
Increased frequency of voiding (colitis, diarrhea)
Compromised neurologic function (peripheral
nerve impairment, spinal cord disease, brain
tumor, encephalitis, infection, degenerative brain
disorders)
Joint pain
Sensory decline
Cognitive dysfunction

*Urinary House Soiling*

Diseases causing polyuria (e.g., renal disease, hyperadrenocorticism, diabetes, pyometra)
Increased urinary frequency (urinary tract infection/
inflammation, urolithiasis, bladder tumors, prostatitis, abdominal masses)
Drugs causing polyuria (e.g., corticosteroids)
Impaired bladder control (peripheral nerve disease,
spinal cord disease, brain tumor, encephalitis, infection, degenerative brain disorders)
Urethral incompetence

Anatomic problems
Urethral sphincter mechanism incompetence
(estrogen-responsive incontinence)
Cognitive dysfunction

### BEHAVIORAL CAUSES

Inadequate training
Submissive urination
Excitement urination
Marking
Separation anxiety
Management-related problems
Location or surface preference

## Cats

### MEDICAL CAUSES

*Fecal House Soiling*

Increased volume of feces (maldigestion, malabsorption, high-fiber diets)
Increased frequency of voiding (colitis, diarrhea, inflammatory bowel disease)
Compromised neurologic function (peripheral nerve impairment, spinal cord disease, brain tumor, encephalitis, infection, degenerative brain disorders)
Joint pain
Anal sacculitis
Obstipation/constipation
Hyperthyroidism
Neoplasia
Cognitive dysfunction

*Urinary House Soiling*

Diseases causing polyuria (e.g., renal disease, hyperadrenocorticism, diabetes, pyometra)
Increased urinary frequency (FLUTD, urolithiasis, idiopathic cystitis)
Impaired bladder control (peripheral nerve disease, spinal cord disease, brain tumor, encephalitis, infection, degenerative brain disorders)
Joint pain, disc disease
Hyperthyroidism
Neoplasia
Anatomic problems
Cognitive dysfunction

### BEHAVIORAL CAUSES

*Litterbox Aversion*

Aversive disorder (deodorant, ammonia)
Inadequate cleaning

Discomfort during elimination (FLUTD, constipation, diarrhea, arthritis)

Unacceptable litter (texture, depth, odor, plastic liner)

Unacceptable box (too small, sides too high, covered)

Disciplined, medicated, or frightened in box

*Location Aversion*

Too much traffic

Traumatic/fearful experience in area

*Other*

Location preference

Surface preference

Anxiety (owner absence, high cat density, moving, new furniture, inappropriate punishment, teasing, household changes, remodeling in home)

Need for privacy (other pets, anything that makes box less accessible to cat)

*Urine Marking*

Hormones

Temperament

Feline population density

Indirect signaling from other cats (scent on visitor's clothing)

Changes in environment (new roommate, remodeling home, new furniture and other novel items in home)

Owner absence from home

Lack of owner attention

Inappropriate punishment

## Incontinence, Fecal

### Nonneurologic Disease

#### COLORECTAL DISEASE

Inflammatory bowel disease

Neoplasia

Constipation

#### ANORECTAL DISEASE

Perianal fistula

Neoplasia

Surgery (anal sacculectomy, perianal herniorrhaphy, rectal resection and anastomosis)

#### MISCELLANEOUS

Decreased mentation

Old age

Severe diarrhea

Irritable bowel disease

## Neurologic Disease

### SACRAL SPINAL CORD DISEASE
Discospondylitis
Neoplasia
Degenerative myelopathy
Congenital vertebral malformation
Sacrococcygeal hypoplasia of Manx cats
Sacral fracture
Sacrococcygeal subluxation
Lumbosacral instability
Meningomyelocele
Viral meningomyelitis

### PERIPHERAL NEUROPATHY
Trauma
Penetrating wounds
Repair of perineal hernia
Perineal urethrostomy
Hypothyroidism
Diabetes mellitus
Dysautonomia

## Incontinence, Urinary

### Bladder Distended

#### NEUROGENIC
Lower motor neuron disease (sacral [S1–S3] segments or
    peripheral nerves)
Bladder easily expressed, dribbles urine
Detrusor areflexia with sphincter areflexia
Upper motor neuron disease
Bladder difficult to express; may be associated with
    paresis, paralysis
Detrusor areflexia with sphincter hypertonia
Dysautonomia

#### OBSTRUCTIVE
Reflex dyssynergia (functional obstruction)
Mechanical obstruction (uroliths, tumors, strictures,
    granulomatous urethritis, urethral inflammation,
    prostatic disease, mucoid or crystalline plug [feline])

### Bladder Not Distended

#### DYSURIA/POLLAKIURIA ABSENT
Urethral sphincter mechanism incompetence (middle-
    aged to older spayed or neutered dogs)
Congenital (ectopic ureters, patent urachus)

### DYSURIA/POLLAKIURIA PRESENT
Detrusor hyperreflexia/instability (uroliths, urinary tract infection, urethral mass)

## Infertility, Female

### Normal Cycles

Improper breeding management
Infertile male
Elevated diestrual progesterone
- Early embryonic death
- Lesions in tubular system (vagina, uterus, uterine tubes)
- Placental lesions (brucellosis, herpes infection)

Normal diestrual progesterone
- Cystic follicles (ovulation failure)

### Abnormal Cycles

#### ABNORMAL ESTRUS

*Will Not Copulate*
Not in estrus
Inexperience
Partner preference
Vaginal anomaly
Hypothyroidism?

*Prolonged Estrus*
Cystic follicles
Ovarian neoplasia
Exogenous estrogens
Prolonged proestrus

*Short Estrus*
Observation error
Geriatric
Split estrus

#### ABNORMAL INTERESTRUAL INTERVAL

*Prolonged Interval*
Photoperiod (queen)
Pseudopregnant/pregnant (queen)
Normal breed variation
Glucocorticoids (bitch)
Geriatric
Luteal cysts

*Short Interval*
Normal (especially queen)
Ovulation failure (especially queen)

Corpus luteum failure
"Split heat" (bitch)
Exogenous drugs

## Not Cycling

Prepubertal
Ovariohysterectomy (OHV)
Estrus suppressants
Silent heat
Unobserved heat
Photoperiod (queen)
Intersex (bitch)
Ovarian dysgenesis
Hypothyroidism (possibly)
Glucocorticoid excess
Hypothalamic–pituitary disorder
Geriatric
Ovarian neoplasia
Premature ovarian failure

## Infertility, Male

### Inflammatory Ejaculate

Prostatitis
Orchitis
Epididymitis

### Azoospermia

Sperm-rich fraction not collected
Sperm not ejaculated
- Incomplete ejaculation
- Obstruction
- Prostate swelling
Sperm not produced
- Endocrine
- Testicular
- Metabolic

### Abnormal Motility/Morphology

Iatrogenic
Prepubertal
Poor ejaculation
Long abstinence

### Abnormal Libido

Female not in estrus
Behavioral

Pain
Geriatric

## Normal Libido

Improper stud management
Infertile female

## Normal Libido/Abnormal Mating Ability

Orthopedic
Neurologic
Prostatic disease
Penile problem
Prepuce problem

## Joint Swelling

Trauma
Degenerative joint disease
Neoplasia
Inflammatory joint disease—infectious
- Septic (bacterial)
- Fungal arthritis
  - Blastomycosis
  - Coccidioidomycosis
  - Cryptococcosis
- Lyme borreliosis
- Rickettsial arthritis
- Leishmaniasis
- Anaplasmosis
- Mycoplasma
- Bacterial L-form–associated arthritis (cats)
- Viral arthritis (calicivirus infection—kittens, canine distemper virus—dogs)

Inflammatory joint disease—noninfectious
- Nonerosive
- Immune-mediated polyarthritis (idiopathic)
- SLE
- Breed-specific polyarthritis syndromes (Akita, Boxer, Weimaraners, Bernese Mountain Dog, German Shorthaired Pointer, Beagle, Shar-Pei)
- Lymphocytic-plasmacytic synovitis
- Drug reaction (e.g., trimethoprim-sulfadiazine in Doberman Pinschers)
- Chronic infection causing secondary immune-mediated polyarthritis (bacterial, ehrlichiosis, anaplasmosis, Rocky Mountain spotted fever, Lyme borreliosis, heartworm disease)

- Erosive
- Rheumatoid arthritis
- Erosive polyarthritis of Greyhounds
- Feline chronic progressive polyarthritis

## Lameness

### Orthopedic

**TRAUMA**
- Fracture
- Luxation, subluxation
- Toenail trauma
- Bone contusion

**INFECTIOUS**
- Osteomyelitis (bacterial, fungal)
- Bacterial cellulitis
- Septic arthritis
- Tick-borne polyarthritis

**IMMUNE-MEDIATED POLYARTHRITIS**

**DEGENERATIVE**
- Degenerative joint disease
- Cranial cruciate disease
- Hip dysplasia
- Elbow dysplasia

**DEVELOPMENTAL**
- Patellar luxation
- Osteochondrosis
- Panosteitis
- Hypertrophic osteodystrophy
- Avascular necrosis of femoral head
- Nonunited anconeal process
- Bone cysts
- Radial agenesis

**METABOLIC**
- Panosteitis
- Hypertrophic osteodystrophy (HOD)
- Diabetic neuropathy

**NUTRITIONAL**
- Vitamin D deficiency (rickets)

**NEOPLASIA**
- Osteosarcoma, synovial cell sarcoma, soft tissue sarcoma/carcinoma

Multiple myeloma
Metastatic to bone

## Muscles

### TRAUMA
Contusion
Strain
Laceration
Rupture

### INFLAMMATORY
Canine idiopathic polymyositis
Feline idiopathic polymyositis
Dermatomyositis

### INFECTIOUS
Protozoal myositis

## Tendons

### TRAUMA
Laceration
Severance
Avulsion

## Ligaments

### TRAUMA
Rupture
Tear
Hyperextension

## Lymphadenopathy (Lymph Node Enlargement)

### Infiltrative Lymphadenopathies

#### NEOPLASTIC
Primary hemolymphatic (lymphoma, multiple myeloma,
systemic mast cell disease, leukemias, malignant
histiocytosis, lymphomatoid granulomatosis)
Metastatic neoplasia (carcinomas, sarcomas, malignant
melanoma, mast cell tumors)

#### NONNEOPLASTIC
Eosinophilic granuloma complex
Nonneoplastic mast cell infiltration
Extramedullary hematopoiesis

### Proliferative and Inflammatory Lymphadenopathies

#### INFECTIOUS
Bacterial

- Localized bacterial infection
- Septicemia
- Systemic infection (e.g., *Borrelia burgdorferi, Brucella canis, Yersinia pestis, Corynebacterium, Mycobacterium, Nocardia, Streptococcus, Actinomyces, Bartonella Ehrlichia* spp.)
- Contagious streptococcal lymphadenopathy

Parasitic (toxoplasmosis, demodicosis, babesiosis, cytaux-zoonosis, hepatozoonosis, leishmaniasis, trypanoso-miasis, *Neospora caninum*)

Rickettsial (ehrlichiosis, Rocky Mountain spotted fever, anaplasmosis, salmon poisoning)

Viral (FIV, FeLV, FIP, canine viral enteritis, infectious canine hepatitis)

Fungal (blastomyosis, cryptococcosis, histoplasmosis, aspergillosis, coccidioidomycosis, phaeohyphomycosis, phycomycosis, sporotrichosis, others)

Algal (prototheccosis) *Pneumocystis carinii*

## NONINFECTIOUS

Immune-mediated disorders
- SLE
- Rheumatoid arthritis
- Immune-mediated polyarthritis
- Juvenile cellulitis

Drug reactions

Localized inflammation

Postvaccinal

Dermatopathic lymphadenopathy

Idiopathic
- Distinctive peripheral lymph node hyperplasia
- Plexiform vascularization of lymph nodes

## Melena

### Ingested Blood

Oral lesions
Nasopharyngeal lesions
Pulmonary lesions
Diet

### Parasitism

Hookworms, protozoa

### Neoplasia

Adenocarcinoma

Lymphoma
Leiomyoma or leiomyosarcoma
Mast cell tumor
Gastrinoma
Nasal or oral tumor

## Upper Gastrointestinal Inflammation

Acute gastritis
Gastroduodenal ulceration/erosion
Hemorrhagic gastroenteritis
Inflammatory bowel disease
Foreign body
Esophagitis

## Infection

Campylobacter
*Clostridium perfringens*
*Salmonella*
*Parvovirus*
*Neorickettsia helminthoeca* (salmon poisoning)
*Histoplasma*
*Pythium*
*Helicobacter*

## Drugs

NSAIDs
Glucocorticoids
Tyrosine kinase inhibitors

## Miscellaneous

Pancreatitis
Liver failure
Renal failure
Hypoadrenocorticism
GI ischemia (shock, volvulus, intussusception)
Arteriovenous fistula
Polyps
Coagulopathies (thrombocytopenia, factor deficiencies, rodenticide toxicity, DIC)

## Muscle Wasting

See **Cachexia and Muscle Wasting**

## Nasal Discharge

See **Sneezing and Nasal Discharge**

## Nystagmus

### Peripheral Vestibular Disease

Horizontal nystagmus; fast phase toward normal side; no change with varying head position

Otitis media/interna

Feline idiopathic vestibular disease

Canine geriatric vestibular disease

Neoplasia

Feline nasopharyngeal polyp in middle ear

Granuloma

Trauma (iatrogenic secondary to ear cleaning)

Ototoxic drugs

Neuropathy (hypothyroid, cranial nerve VIII disease)

Congenital (German Shepherd, English Cocker Spaniel, Doberman Pinscher, Smooth-Haired Fox Terrier, Siamese, Burmese, Tonkinese)

### Central Vestibular Disease

Horizontal, vertical, or rotary nystagmus; direction may change with varying head position. Disconjugate nystagmus (each eye oscillates in a different direction) also indicates central lesion.

Trauma/hemorrhage

Infectious inflammatory disease

Viral (canine distemper virus, FIP)

Rickettsial (Rocky Mountain spotted fever, ehrlichiosis)

Fungal (cryptococcosis)

Toxoplasmosis

Neosporosis

Granulomatous meningoencephalitis

Neoplasia

Vascular infarct

Thiamine deficiency

Metronidazole toxicity

Toxic (lead, hexachlorophene)

Degenerative diseases (storage diseases, neuronopathies, demyelinating diseases)

Hydrocephalus

Anomaly (caudal occipital malformation syndrome in Cavalier King Charles Spaniels)

Head trauma

## Obesity

### Causes

Excessive feeding
Malnutrition
High-carbohydrate diet (especially cats)
Lack of exercise
Inactivity (indoor lifestyle, middle age)
Orthopedic disease
Neutering?
Genetic predisposition
Hypothyroidism
Hyperadrenocorticism
Hyperinsulinism
Acromegaly
Hypopituitarism
Hypothalamic dysfunction
Drugs (glucocorticoids, progestogens, phenobarbital,
primidone)

### Health Risks

Degenerative joint disease
Cruciate ligament disease
Hip dysplasia
Traumatic joint disease
Intervertebral disk disease
Dyspnea (Pickwickian syndrome)
Heat intolerance
Exercise intolerance
Diabetes mellitus (insulin resistance)
Hepatic lipidosis (cats)
Pancreatitis
Dystocia
Urinary tract disease
Skin fold dermatoses
Increased anesthetic risk

## Oliguria

See **Anuria and Oliguria**

## Pallor

### Anemia

#### REGENERATIVE ANEMIA
Immune-mediated hemolytic anemia (extravascular,
intravascular)

Erythrocytic parasites (*Bartonella, Babesia, Cytauxzoon* spp.)

Fragmentation (DIC, heartworm disease, hemangiosarcoma, vasculitis, hemolytic uremic syndrome, diabetes mellitus)

Pyruvate kinase deficiency

Phosphofructokinase deficiency

Feline porphyria

Copper toxicity

Neonatal isoerythrolysis

Oxidative injury (onions, acetaminophen, zinc, benzocaine, mothballs, phenazopyridine)

Blood loss (external blood loss, blood loss to a body cavity, coagulopathies, endoparasites, GI blood loss)

### NONREGENERATIVE ANEMIA

Anemia of chronic disease

Anemia from renal failure

FeLV

Endocrine (mild anemia associated with hypoadrenocorticism, hypothyroidism)

Myeloaplasia/aplastic anemia (FeLV infection, ehrlichiosis, trimethoprim-sulfa, estrogen toxicity, phenylbutazone, chemotherapy, chloramphenicol)

Myelodysplasia

Myeloproliferative and lymphoproliferative disorders

Myelofibrosis

## Shock

### CARDIOGENIC

Decreased ventricular function

- Dilated cardiomyopathy
- Myocarditis
- Myocardial infarction

Compromised ventricular filling

- Hypertrophic cardiomyopathy
- Cardiac tamponade

Severe endocardiosis

Outflow obstruction

- Intracardiac tumors
- Aortic stenosis
- Hypertrophic obstructive cardiomyopathy
- Heartworm disease
- Thrombosis
- Severe arrhythmia

**NONCARDIOGENIC**

Trauma

Hypovolemia

- Severe blood loss
- Dehydration
- Hypoadrenocorticism

Disruptions in blood flow

- Sepsis and endotoxemia
- Hypotension
- Anaphylaxis

## Panting

### Differential Diagnosis of Panting

Elevated ambient temperature
Exercise-induced hyperthermia
Excessive/matted coat
Obesity
Fever
Pain
Anxiety/nervousness
Glucocorticoid therapy
Hyperadrenocorticism
Hyperthyroidism
Cardiac disease, tachyarrhythmia
Feline bronchial disease
Narcotic administration
Hypocalcemia
Pheochromocytoma
Brain disease

## Papules and Pustules

Bacterial pyoderma (papules and pustules)
Demodicosis (papules and pustules)
Dermatophytosis (rare papules, uncommon pustules)
Sarcoptic mange (papules, no pustules)
Cheyletiellosis (rare papules, no pustules)
Otoacariasis (rare papules, no pustules)
Trombiculosis (papules, rare pustules)
Hypersensitivity (papules, rare pustules)
Pemphigus (papules and pustules)
Early stage neoplasia (papules, no pustules)

## Paresis and Paralysis

### Upper Motor Neuron

Tetraparesis or hemiparesis
- Severe forebrain lesion
- Brain stem lesion
- First to fifth cervical (C1–C5) spinal lesion

Paraparesis or rear limb monoparesis
- Third thoracic to third lumbar (T3–L3) spinal lesion

### Lower Motor Neuron

Tetraparesis
Generalized lower motor neuron disease
- Flaccid paresis/paralysis
- Acute polyradiculoneuritis/"Coonhound paralysis"
- Tick paralysis
- Botulism
- Myasthenia gravis
- Toxicants
- Coral snake
- Black widow spider
- Herbicides (2,4-D)
- Macadamia nuts

Paraparesis
- Fourth lumbar to second sacral (L4–S2) spinal lesion

Hemiparesis with lower motor neuron forelimb
- Sixth cervical to second thoracic (C6–T2) spinal lesion

Aortic thromboembolism
Degenerative myelopathy
Monoparesis
Peripheral nerve lesion

## Petechiae and Ecchymoses

### Thrombocytopenia

#### INCREASED PLATELET DESTRUCTION
Immune-mediated thrombocytopenia
SLE
Heartworm disease

#### DECREASED PLATELET PRODUCTION
*Bone Marrow Suppression*
Infectious disease (ehrlichiosis, babesiosis, Rocky
Mountain spotted fever, leishmaniasis, FeLV, FIV)
Neoplasia
Drug reactions
Myeloproliferative disease

Virus-associated myelodysplasia
Estrogen toxicity

### CONSUMPTION OF PLATELETS
DIC
Vasculitis

### SEQUESTRATION OF PLATELETS (UNLIKELY TO CAUSE CLINICAL SIGNS)
Splenomegaly
Hepatomegaly
Endotoxemia

## Thrombopathia

### INHERITED
Chédiak -Higashi syndrome of Persian cats
Thrombasthenia of Otterhound, Great Pyrenees
Delta storage-pool disease of American Cocker Spaniel,
Other thrombopathies: Bassett Hound, German
Shepherd, Greater Swiss Mountain Dog, Pug, Spitz,
Gray collies with cyclic hematopoiesis, cats

### ACQUIRED
Drugs (aspirin, other NSAIDs, acepromazine, cephalothin,
carprofen, hydroxyethyl starch)
Uremia
Liver disease
Dysproteinemias

### VON WILLEBRAND DISEASE
Lack of von Willebrand factor leads to impaired platelet
adhesion

## Vascular Purpura

Vasculitis secondary to infectious, inflammatory, or
immune-mediated diseases, neoplasia, drug reaction, or
hyperadrenocorticism

## Pollakiuria

See **Stranguria, Dysuria, and Pollakiuria**

## Polyphagia

### Primary Polyphagia

Destruction of satiety center (mass lesion, trauma,
infection/inflammation)
Psychogenic/gluttony
Stress
Introduction of more palatable diet

## Secondary Polyphagia

Physiologically increased metabolic rate (cold temperature, pregnancy, lactation, growth, exercise)

Pathologically increased metabolic rate (hyperthyroidism, infection, neoplasia)

Decreased energy supply (diabetes mellitus, exocrine pancreatic insufficiency, infiltrative bowel disease, parasites, lymphangiectasia)

Decreased intake (low-calorie diet, hypoglycemia, megaesophagus)

Unknown (hyperadrenocorticism, portosystemic shunt/ hepatoencephalopathy, SARDS)

## Drug-Induced Polyphagia

Glucocorticoids, phenobarbital, antihistamines, progestins, benzodiazepines, cyproheptadine, mirtazapine

### Polyuria and Polydipsia

Renal insufficiency or failure
Diabetes mellitus
Hyperadrenocorticism (Cushing syndrome)
Lower urinary tract disease
- Infection
- Urolithiasis
- Neoplasia
- Anatomic problem
- Neurologic problem
Pyometra
Hypercalcemia
Hypoadrenocorticism (Addison disease)
Pyelonephritis
Ethylene glycol intoxication
Hypokalemia
Iatrogenic (corticosteroids, diuretics, anticonvulsants)
Hyperthyroidism
Hepatic insufficiency
Postobstructive
Diabetes insipidus
- Central
- Renal
Psychogenic drinking
Renal glycosuria

## Preputial Discharge

### Mucopurulent

- Balanoposthitis
- Prostatitis
- Penile neoplasia
- Foreign body
- Orchitis/epididymitis
- Persistent penile frenulum
- Hypospadias

### Serosanguinous

- Benign prostatic hyperplasia
- Balanoposthitis
- Prostatitis
- Urethral prolapse
- Penile/urethral trauma
- Penile/urethral uroliths
- Penile neoplasia
- Hemorrhagic diathesis
- Foreign body

## Pruritus

### Allergy

Flea allergy
Atopic dermatitis
Food allergy/intolerance
Contact dermatitis
Mosquitobite hypersensitivity
Eosinophilic plaque (cats)

### Parasites

Flea infestation
Scabies
Pediculosis (lice)
Cheyletiellosis
Chiggers
Cutaneous larval migrans
Demodicosis (often not pruritic)
Otodectic acariasis
Notoedres acariasis

### Infectious Agents

Pyoderma
*Malassezia* dermatitis
Dermatophytosis

## Behavioral

Acral lick dermatosis
Psychogenic alopecia

## Immune-Mediated

Pemphigus foliaceus

## Drug Eruption

## Miscellaneous

Cornification defects
Superficial necrolytic dermatitis
Tail dock neuroma
Rhabditic dermatitis
Calcinosis cutis
Cutaneous lymphoma

## Ptyalism (Excessive Salivation)

## Oral Cavity Disease

Oral trauma (tooth fractures, mandibular fractures, maxillary fractures, temporomandibular joint [TMJ] luxation)
Severe periodontal disease
Oral masses (neoplasia, granuloma, eosinophilic granuloma)
Abscesses
Stomatitis (toxins, infections, immune-mediated disease, immunologic, or nutritional deficiency)
Glossitis (chemical or environmental irritants, viral infections, uremia, immune-mediated disease, tumors)
Oral ulcers/burns
Faucitis (cats)
Mucocutaneous junction lesions
Foreign body
Developmental (severe brachygnathism, lip fold pyoderma)
Conformational drooling

## Oral Cavity Normal

Drugs and toxins (bitter taste; insecticides such as organophosphates, pyrethrins, and D-limonene; caustic chemicals; cannabis/marijuana; poisonous toads and salamanders)
Nausea
Hepatic encephalopathy/portosystemic shunt
Seizures
Space-occupying lesions in pharynx

Cranial nerve (CN) deficits (CN V: inability to close mouth; CN VII: inability to move lip; CNs X, XI, and XII: loss of gag lesion and inability to swallow)

Neuromuscular (myasthenia gravis, temporal or masseter muscle atrophy, tetanus)

Esophagitis/megaesophagus

Rabies virus

Dysphagia

Behavior (associated with food [Pavlovian], contentment/ mood in cats when purring, pain)

Salivary gland hypersecretion

## Pulse Abnormalities

- Hyperkinetic pulse
    1. Anemia
    2. Hyperthyroidism
    3. Increased sympathetic tone
    4. Bradyarrhythmias
    5. Aortic insufficiency
    6. Patent ductus arteriosus
    7. Pregnancy
    8. Aorticopulmonary window
    9. Arteriovenous fistula/anastomosis
- Hypokinetic pulse
    1. Hypovolemia
    2. Reduced systolic function
    3. Aortic/subaortic stenosis
    4. Dynamic left ventricular outflow tract obstruction
- Decrease in pulse volume with inspiration
    1. Pericardial effusion with cardiac tamponade
    2. Exaggerated variation in intrapleural pressure (airway obstruction)
- Pulse deficits
    1. Atrial fibrillation
    2. Atrial/supraventricular premature complexes
    3. Ventricular premature complexes
    4. Pulsus alternans (alternating normal pulse and pulse deficits with myocardial failure)
- Irregular pulse rhythm
    1. Sinus arrhythmia (slow)
    2. Atrial fibrillation
    3. Atrial/supraventricular premature complexes (rapid)
    4. Ventricular premature complexes (rapid)
    5. Second-degree atrioventricular (AV) block (slow)
- Regional pulse variation
    1. Arterial thromboembolism

## Regurgitation

### Esophageal Disease

Megaesophagus (primary or secondary)
Esophagitis
Mechanical obstruction (foreign body, vascular ring
   anomaly, stricture, neoplasia)

### Alimentary Disorders

Pyloric outflow obstruction
Gastric dilatation/volvulus
Hiatal hernia

### Neuropathies

Peripheral neuropathy (polyradiculitis, polyneuritis, lead
   poisoning, giant cell axonal neuropathy)
CNS (brain stem lesion, neoplastic, traumatic, distemper)
Dysautonomia

### Neuromuscular Junction Abnormalities

Myasthenia gravis (focal or generalized)
Tetanus
Botulism
Acetylcholinesterase toxicity

### Immune-Mediated Disorders

SLE
Polymyositis
Dermatomyositis

### Endocrine Disease

Hypothyroidism
Hypoadrenocorticism

### Infectious

Spirocercosis
*Pythium insidiosum*

### Neoplasia

Thoracic neoplasia (thymoma)

## Restlessness

### Causes of Restless Behaviors in Dogs and Cats

#### NORMAL BEHAVIOR

Discomfort from pollakiuria or tenesmus
Periparturient

Estrous

Pseudopregnancy

## EMOTIONAL DISTRESS

Fear/phobia

Stress from altered environment or blindness

Pending natural calamity (e.g., earthquake)

Anxiety

## PAIN

## PHYSIOLOGIC DISTRESS

Shock

Transfusion reaction

Anaphylaxis

Iatrogenic overhydration

Dyspnea

Pheochromocytoma

Overheating

Fever

Pruritus

## INTOXICATION

Drug-induced (antipsychotics, tricyclic antidepressants, selective serotonin reuptake inhibitors, methylxanthines, sympathomimetics, prostaglandins, opioids, metoclopramide, antihistamines [cats], digoxin, salicylates, benzodiazepines [excitatory phase], drug- or anesthesia-induced dysphoria)

Other toxic substances (metaldehyde, pyrethrins, strychnine, nicotine, organophosphates/carbamates, recreational drugs [amphetamine, cocaine], mycotoxins)

## ALTERED MENTATION/ENCEPHALOPATHY

Primary CNS disease (epileptic aura [preictal], tumors, inflammation, rabies/pseudorabies, geriatric cognitive dysfunction)

Metabolic encephalopathies (hepatic encephalopathy, hypoglycemia, hypocalcemia)

## INCREASED METABOLIC RATE

Hyperthyroidism (iatrogenic or spontaneous)

## Reverse Sneezing

Loud inspiratory noise, occurs in paroxysms; initiated by nasopharyngeal irritation

Purpose is to move secretions and foreign material into the oropharynx to be swallowed

Causes include excitement, foreign bodies, nasal mites
(*Pneumonyssus caninum*), viral infections, and epiglottic
entrapment of the soft palate

Often idiopathic, nonprogressive, and common in small dogs
and cats

## Scaling and Crusting

### Bacterial

Superficial folliculitis
Deep pyoderma
Mucocutaneous pyoderma
Pyotraumatic dermatitis

### Fungal

Dermatophytosis
*Malassezia* dermatitis
Deep fungal infection (e.g., blastomycosis, cryptococcosis)

### Parasitic

Fleas
Scabies
Demodicosis
Cheyletiellosis
Notoedric mange
Pediculosis

### Protozoal

Leishmaniasis

### Viral

FeLV

### Allergic

Atopic dermatitis
Food hypersensitivity
Flea-bite hypersensitivity
Military dermatitis

### Endocrine and Metabolic

Hyperadrenocorticism
Hypothyroidism
Necrolytic migratory erythema

### Immune-Mediated

Pemphigus foliaceus
DLE
Erythema multiforme

## Congenital and Hereditary

Primary seborrhea
Ichthyosis
Schnauzer comedo syndrome
Familial canine dermatomyositis

## Keratinization Defects

Secondary seborrhea
Vitamin A–responsive dermatosis
Ear margin dermatosis

## Environmental

Solar dermatitis

## Nutritional

Zinc-responsive dermatosis
Fatty acid deficiency

## Other

Cutaneous lymphoma
Sebaceous adenitis
Otitis externa

## Seizure

### Extracranial Causes

Toxins (e.g., strychnine, chlorinated hydrocarbons, organophosphates, carbamates, lead, ethylene glycol, metaldehyde)
Metabolic disease (e.g., hepatic encephalopathy, hypoglycemia, hypocalcemia)
Hepatic disease
Electrolyte disturbances (e.g., hypernatremia)
Severe uremia
Hyperlipoproteinemia
Hyperviscosity (multiple myeloma, polycythemia)
Hyperosmolality (diabetes mellitus)
Heat stroke
Hypertension
Hyperthyroidism (cats)
Hypothyroidism (dogs)

### Intracranial Causes

See **Part Two**, Section XI: **Differential Diagnosis for Inflammatory Disease of the Nervous System**
Infectious disease

Neoplasia (primary brain tumor, lymphoma, metastatic tumors)

Head trauma/brain scar tissue

Granulomatous meningoencephalitis

Hemorrhage/infarct (renal failure, hypothyroidism, hyperthyroidism, hypertension, septic emboli, neoplasia, coagulopathies, heartworm disease, vasculitis)

Congenital malformations (lissencephaly, hydrocephalus)

Necrotizing meningoencephalitis, necrotizing leukoencephalitis

Degenerative diseases (metabolic storage diseases, leukodystrophies, hypomyelination disorders, spongy disorders)

## Idiopathic Epilepsy (Primary Epileptic Seizures)
## Epilepsy

## Sneezing and Nasal Discharge

## Nasal and Upper Respiratory Disease

### INFECTIOUS

Viral: feline herpesvirus, calicivirus, canine distemper virus

Bacterial: *Mycoplasma* spp., *Bordetella bronchiseptica*

Fungal: *Aspergillus, Cryptococcus, Rhinosporidium, Penicillium* spp.

Parasitic: *Pneumonyssus caninum* (nasal mite), *Eucoleus boehmi* (formerly *Capillaria* spp.), *Cuterebra* spp., *Linguatula spp.*

### INFLAMMATORY

Allergic rhinitis

Lymphocytic-plasmacytic rhinitis

Acquired nasopharyngeal stenosis

Nasopharyngeal polyps

Polypoid rhinitis

### NEOPLASIA

Adenocarcinoma, squamous cell carcinoma

Fibrosarcoma, osteosarcoma, chondrosarcoma

Lymphoma, transmissible venereal tumor, neuroendocrine carcinoma

### FOREIGN BODY

### CONGENITAL

Cleft palate

Ciliary dyskinesia

Nasopharyngeal stenosis

Choanal atresia

### DENTAL DISEASE
Tooth root abscess
Oronasal fistula

### TRAUMA

### VASCULAR MALFORMATION

## Systemic Disease

### INFECTIOUS
Canine distemper virus
Canine infectious tracheobronchitis
Pneumonia

### HYPERTENSION
Hyperthyroidism
Hyperadrenocorticism
Renal disease
Pheochromocytoma
Hypothyroidism
Acromegaly
Polycythemia
Diabetes mellitus
Overhydration

### COAGULOPATHIES
Thrombocytopenia
Rocky Mountain spotted fever
Thrombocytopathia
von Willebrand disease
Factor deficiencies
Congenital (hemophilia A, B, others)
Acquired (vitamin K rodenticide toxicity, DIC, hepatic
  failure)

### VASCULITIS
Toxic
Inflammatory
Immune-mediated (SLE)
Neoplastic
Infectious (ehrlichiosis, FIP, Rocky Mountain spotted
  fever, leishmaniasis)

### HYPERVISCOSITY
Multiple myeloma
Lymphoma
IgM (Waldenström) macroglobulinemia
Chronic lymphocytic leukemia
Ehrlichiosis

Amyloidosis
Plasma cell leukemia
FIP (rare)

## Stertor and Stridor

### Stertor

Snoring or snorting associated with partial nasal or naso-pharyngeal obstruction

#### INTRANASAL DISORDERS
Congenital deformities
Masses
Exudates
Stenotic nares
Clotted blood

### Pharyngeal Disease

Brachycephalic airway syndrome
Elongated soft palate
Nasopharyngeal polyp
Foreign body
Neoplasia
Abscess
Granuloma
Extraluminal mass

### Stridor

High-pitched wheeze caused by air turbulence in upper airway associated with laryngeal disease or narrowing of extrathoracic trachea

#### LARYNGEAL DISEASE
Neoplasia
Polyps (nasopharyngeal)
Laryngeal paralysis
Laryngeal trauma
Foreign body
Acute laryngitis/obstructive laryngitis
Brachycephalic airway syndrome
Rhinitis
Coagulopathy

#### EXTRATHORACIC TRACHEAL DISEASE
Neoplasia
Foreign body
Extrathoracic collapsing trachea
Extraluminal mass

## Stranguria, Dysuria, and Pollakiuria

### Stranguria/Pollakiuria

#### SMALL BLADDER
Cystitis
- Infectious agents
- Idiopathic cystitis (cats)
- Chemically induced cystitis (cyclophosphamide)
- Polypoid cystitis

Detrusor hyperspasticity
Urethritis
Urethral mass

#### LARGE BLADDER
Lower urinary tract obstruction
- Functional
- Mechanical

### Urinary Retention

#### EASY CATHETERIZATION
*Normal Neurologic Examination*
Cystic calculi or mass
Detrusor areflexia from overdistension
Reflex dyssynergia

*Abnormal Neurologic Examination*
Detrusor areflexia with sphincter areflexia (lower motor neuron)
Detrusor areflexia with sphincter hypertonia (upper motor neuron)
Dysautonomia

#### DIFFICULT CATHETERIZATION
Urethral spasm
Urethral calculi
Urethral stricture
Urethral neoplasia
Transitional cell carcinoma
Granulomatous urethritis
Urethral inflammation
Prostatic disease (benign prostatic hyperplasia, neoplasia)
Mucoid or crystalline plug (cats)

## Stomatitis

Infectious disease
- FIV
- FeLV

- Feline syncytium-forming virus
- Feline calicivirus
- Feline herpesvirus
- FIP
- Bartonellosis
- Canine distemper virus
- Feline panleukopenia virus
- Candidiasis

Immunosuppressive disease
Feline eosinophilic granuloma complex
Idiopathic feline chronic gingivitis/stomatitis
Immune-mediated disease

- SLE
- Bullous (pemphigus) disease
- Idiopathic vasculitis
- Toxic epidermal necrolysis
- Ulcerative gingivitis/stomatitis of Maltese
- Sjögren-like syndrome

Uremic stomatitis
Radiation-induced

## Stunted Growth

### Small Stature and Poor Body Condition

Nutritional (poor-quality feed, underfeeding)
Gastrointestinal (parasitism, food intolerance/allergy, inflammatory bowel disease, exocrine pancreatic insufficiency, obstruction)
Esophageal disease (congenital myasthenia gravis, megaesophagus, vascular ring anomaly most commonly persistent right aortic arch)
Cardiac (dog: most commonly subaortic stenosis, patent ductus arteriosus, pulmonic stenosis) (cat: most commonly ventricular septal defect, AV valve dysplasia)
Systemic disease (metabolic/infectious: kidney disease, liver disease like portal systemic shunt, glycogen storage disease, mucopolysaccharidosis, respiratory infections like bacterial pneumonia, GI infections)
Endocrine (diabetes mellitus, hypoadrenocorticism, diabetes insipidus, juvenile hypoparathyroidism)

### Small Stature and Good Body Condition

- Bone growth (osteochondrodystrophy: disproportionate dwarfism)
- Endocrine
  1. Disproportionate dwarfism: congenital hypothyroidism

**2.** Proportionate dwarfism: hyposomatotropism (growth hormone deficiency), hyperadrenocorticism (rare)

## Stupor and Coma
### Increased Intracranial Pressure

Encephalitis
Meningitis
Neoplasia
Granulomas
Abscess
Vascular events (hemorrhage, embolism, ischemia)
Trauma
Underlying metabolic injury (e.g., hypertension)
Developmental (hydrocephalus, storage diseases)

### Systemic Infections

Rabies
FIP
Canine distemper
Fungal
Parasitic

### Cerebral Edema

Vasogenic (brain masses that lead to breakdown of blood–brain barrier)
Cytotoxic (hypoxia, neuroglycopenia)
Interstitial (hydrocephalus)

### Herniation of Brain Tissue

Caudal transtentorial herniation
Foramen magnum herniation

### Extracranial Causes

Hypoglycemia
Hypernatremia
Hyponatremia
Diabetic ketoacidosis
Uremic encephalopathy
Severe hypothyroidism (myxedema coma)
Heat stroke
Toxins
Hepatic disease
Hyperadrenocorticism
Erythrocytosis
Hyperglobulinemia

## Syncope

### Normal Cerebral Perfusion

Severe hypoxemia
Hypoglycemia

### Cerebral Hypoperfusion

#### NORMOTENSION

Cerebrovascular disease
Cerebral vasoconstriction
Tussive syncope

#### SYSTEMIC HYPOTENSION

*Decreased Cardiac Output*

Loss of Preload

Cardiac tamponade, atrial ball thrombi, atrial myxoma, AV valve stenosis, hypovolemia, diuretics

Obstruction to Flow

Aortic and subaortic stenosis, pulmonic stenosis, pulmonary hypertension, pulmonary thromboembolism, outflow tract tumors, myocardial infarction, hypertrophic and restrictive cardiomyopathy, systolic anterior motion of mitral valve, infundibular stenosis, heartworm disease, masses obstructing flow

Arrhythmias

Bradyarrhythmias: sick sinus syndrome, third-degree AV block, persistent atrial standstill, β-blockers, calcium channel blockers
Tachyarrhythmias: atrial fibrillation, atrial tachycardia, AV reentrant tachycardia, ventricular tachycardia, drug-induced proarrhythmia, torsades de pointes

Loss of Vascular Resistance

Drug therapy: angiotensin-converting enzyme (ACE) inhibitors, β-blockers, calcium channel blockers, hydralazine, nitrates, phenothiazines
Reflex syncope (neurally mediated): orthostatic, postexertion, micturition, defecation, cough, emotional distress, pain, carotid sinus hypersensitivity
Autonomic nervous system disease: primary or secondary (diabetes mellitus, paraneoplastic, chronic renal failure, autoimmune disease, amyloidosis)
Cyanotic heart disease (tetralogy of Fallot, reversed shunt)

## Tachycardia, Sinus

Anxiety/fear
Excitement
Exercise pain
Hyperthyroidism
Heart failure
Hyperthermia/fever
Anemia
Hypoxia
Shock
Hypotension
Sepsis
Drugs (anticholinergics, sympathomimetics)
Toxicity (e.g., chocolate, amphetamines, theophylline)
Electric shock
Any cause of high sympathetic tone

## Tenesmus and Dyschezia

### Colonic or Rectal Obstruction

Constipation
Pelvic fracture
Rectal neoplasia
Anal sac neoplasia
Extraluminal neoplasia
Prostatomegaly
Perineal hernia
Pelvic canal mass
Rectal granuloma
Rectal foreign body
Rectal stricture
Perianal gland tumors
Pseudocoprostasis

### Perineal Inflammation or Pain

Anal sacculitis
Perianal fistula
Perianal abscess/abscessed anal sac

### Rectal Inflammation or Pain

Rectal tumor/polyp
Proctitis
Histoplasmosis
Pythiosis

## Colonic Inflammation

Idiopathic colitis
Bacterial
Fungal
Parasites
Dietary indiscretion
Inflammatory bowel disease
Neoplasia

## Tremor

### Physiologic Tremor

Hypothermia (shiver)
Heavy exercise/exhaustion
Fear
Pain
Weakness

### Pathologic Tremor

Metabolic disorders (renal disease, hypoglycemia, hypocalcemia, hypoadrenocorticism, hepatic encephalopathy)
Intracranial infectious disease (*Neospora caninum*, cerebellar hypoplasia secondary to intrauterine panleukopenia infection)
Intracranial disease (fibrinoid leukodystrophy, neuraxonal dystrophy, Labrador Retriever axonopathy, spongiform encephalopathy, neuronal abiotrophies, subacute necrotizing encephalopathy, lysosomal storage diseases)
Hind end tremor (intervertebral disk herniation, tumors, discospondylitis, nerve root compression, peripheral neuropathies)
Corticoid-responsive tremor syndrome (formerly "white shaker disease")
Myasthenia gravis
Cerebellar malformation
Hypomyelination
Spongy degeneration
Tremorgenic toxins (mycotoxins penitrem A and roquefortine produced by *Penicillium* spp. growing on spoiled foods; metaldehyde, hexachlorophene, bromethalin, organophosphates, carbamates, pyrethroids, xanthines, macadamia nuts, strychnine, trazodone, fluoxetine, diphenhydramine, blue-green algae)
Idiopathic head tremor in Doberman Pinschers and Bulldogs
Idiopathic tremor of hind legs of geriatric dogs

## Urine, Discolored

### Red, Pink, Red-Brown, Red-Orange, or Orange

Hematuria
Hemoglobinuria
Myoglobinuria
Porphyrinuria
Pyuria

### Orange-Yellow

Highly concentrated urine
Urobilin
Bilirubin

### Yellow-Brown or Green-Brown

Bile pigments

### Brown to Black

Melanin
Methemoglobin
Myoglobin
Bile pigments

### Brown

Methemoglobin
Melanin

### Colorless

Dilute urine

### Milky White

Lipid
Pyuria
Crystals

### Pale Yellow

Normal
Dilute urine

## Urticaria/Angioedema

### Immediate Hypersensitivity Reaction

Insect bites/stings
Food
Drugs/vaccines
Airborne allergens (atopy)

## Nonimmunologic Stimulus by Irritant

Weeds
Insects
Physical stimuli (cold, heat, sunlight)
Psychogenic stimuli

## Vision Loss, Sudden

See **Blindness**

## Vomiting

### Gastric Disease

Gastritis
Parasites
Foreign body
Obstruction
Ulceration
Neoplasia
Dilatation/volvulus
*Helicobacter* infection
Gastric ulcer
Hiatal hernia
Motility disorders
Pyloric stenosis
Gastric antral mucosal hypertrophy

### Small Intestinal Disease

Parasites
Inflammatory bowel disease
Foreign body
Bacterial overgrowth/enteritis
Acute hemorrhagic diarrhea syndrome (formerly hemorrhagic
    gastroenteritis)
Neoplasia
Viral enteritis (parvovirus, canine distemper virus)
Intussusception
Nonneoplastic infiltrative disease (e.g., pythiosis)

### Large Intestinal Disease

Colitis
Obstipation
Parasites

### Dietary

Indiscretion
Intolerance
Allergy

## Drugs

Cancer chemotherapeutic agents
Antibiotics (especially erythromycin, tetracycline)
NSAIDs
Cardiac glycosides
Apomorphine
Xylazine
Penicillamine

## Extraalimentary Tract Disease

Peritonitis
Pancreatitis
Hepatobiliary disease
Neoplasia
Uremia
Diabetes mellitus/ketoacidosis
Hypercalcemia
Hyperthyroidism
Hypoadrenocorticism
Hepatic disease
Hepatic encephalopathy
Septicemia/endotoxemia
Pyometra
Acid–base disorders
Electrolyte disorders
Hypertriglyceridemia
Gastrinoma (Zollinger-Ellison syndrome)
Mastocytosis
Motion sickness

## Intoxicants

Numerous inorganic, organic, and plant toxins can cause GI
irritation and vomiting.

## Neurologic Disease

Epilepsy, tumor, meningitis, increased intracranial pressure,
dysautonomia, vestibular disease

### Vulvar Discharge

## Serosanguinous Vaginal Discharge

### INTACT
Physiologic estrogen influence (proestrus)
Prolonged estrogen duration (ovarian neoplasia, cystic
ovarian follicles, failure to ovulate, exogenous estrogen, portosystemic shunt, pituitary hypofunction)

Absence of estrogen influence (endometriosis, neoplasia of urogenital tract, subinvolution of placental sites, trauma, hemorrhagic diathesis, vaginal foreign body)

**AFTER OVARIOHYSTERECTOMY**

- Estrogen influence (remnant ovarian syndrome, exogenous estrogen)
- Absence of estrogen influence (stump endometritis secondary to presence of remnant ovarian syndrome with progesterone influence, uterine stump hemorrhage post-OVH, neoplasia of urogenital tract, trauma, hemorrhagic diathesis, vaginal foreign body)

## Mucopurulent Vaginal Discharge

**INTACT**

Physiologic (onset of diestrus, pregnancy [clear mucus])
Pathologic (pyometra, endometritis postestrum or postpartum, abortion, vestibulitis/vaginitis, neoplasia, vaginal foreign body)

**AFTER OVARIOHYSTERECTOMY**

Vaginitis, stump endometritis secondary to presence of remnant ovarian syndrome with progesterone influence, hypersecretion of vaginal mucosa, neoplasia, vaginal foreign body)

## Weakness

Very nonspecific clinical sign of disease
Metabolic disease
Inflammation
- Infectious disease (bacterial, viral, fungal, rickettsial, protozoal, parasitic)
- Immune-mediated disease
Fever
Electrolyte disorders
- Hypokalemia, hyperkalemia, hyponatremia, hypernatremia, hypocalcemia, hypomagnesemia
Acid–base disorders
Abdominal effusion
Anemia
Poor oxygen delivery
Endocrine disease
- Diabetes mellitus, hypothyroidism, hypoadrenocorticism, hyperadrenocorticism, hypoglycemia, hyperparathyroidism, hypoparathyroidism, pheochromocytoma

Cardiovascular disease
Hypotension, hypertension
Respiratory disease
Skeletal disease
Neuromuscular disease
- Brain disease (encephalitis, cerebrovascular accidents, space-occupying lesions, vestibular disease, idiopathic epilepsy)
- Spinal cord diseases
- Neuropathies (e.g., polyradiculoneuritis, myasthenia gravis, developmental disorders, toxoplasmosis, neosporosis)

Neoplasia
Cachexia
Physical and psychologic stress
Malnutrition
Drugs
- Anticonvulsants, antihistamines, glucocorticoids, tranquilizers, narcotics, cardiac drugs

Toxins
Pain

## Weight Gain

See **Obesity**

## Weight Loss

See **Cachexia and Muscle Wasting**

# PART TWO

# SYSTEMIC APPROACH TO DIFFERENTIAL DIAGNOSIS

## Mechanisms of Disease

### DAMNIT-VP Scheme

**D**   Degenerative, developmental
**A**   Anomalous
**M**   Metabolic, malformation
**N**   Neoplastic, nutritional
**I**    Infectious, inflammatory, immune, iatrogenic, inherited, idiopathic
**T**   Traumatic, toxic
**V**   Vascular
**P**   Parasitic

# Cardiopulmonary Disorders

## Arrhythmias

### Differential Diagnosis

#### SLOW, IRREGULAR RHYTHMS
Sinus bradyarrhythmias
Sinus arrest
Sick sinus syndrome
High-grade second-degree atrioventricular (AV) block

#### SLOW, REGULAR RHYTHMS
Sinus bradycardia
Complete AV block with ventricular escape rhythm
Atrial standstill with ventricular escape rhythm

#### FAST, IRREGULAR RHYTHMS
Atrial or supraventricular premature contractions
Paroxysmal atrial or supraventricular tachycardia
Atrial flutter

Atrial fibrillation
Ventricular premature contractions
Paroxysmal ventricular tachycardia

## FAST, REGULAR RHYTHMS
Sinus tachycardia
Sustained supraventricular tachycardia
Sustained ventricular tachycardia

## NORMAL, IRREGULAR RHYTHMS (REQUIRE NO TREATMENT)
Respiratory sinus arrhythmia
Wandering pacemaker

# Arterial Thromboembolism
## Clinical Findings

### ACUTE LIMB PARESIS
Posterior paresis ("saddle" thrombus: most common
    presentation)
Monoparesis (right subclavian artery thrombus; second
    most common presentation in cats)
Intermittent claudication
Severe limb pain
Cool distal limbs
Cyanotic nail beds
Arterial pulse absent
Contracture of affected muscles
Vocalization (pain, distress)

### RENAL INFARCTION
Renal pain
Acute renal failure

### SPLENIC INFARCTION
Lethargy
Anorexia
Vomiting
Diarrhea

### MESENTERIC INFARCTION
Abdominal pain
Vomiting
Diarrhea

### CEREBRAL INFARCTION
Neurologic deficits
Seizures
Sudden death

## SIGNS OF HEART FAILURE
Systolic murmur
Gallop rhythm
Tachypnea/dyspnea
Weakness/lethargy
Anorexia
Arrhythmias
Hypothermia
Cardiomegaly
Effusions
Pulmonary edema

## HEMATOLOGIC AND BIOCHEMICAL ABNORMALITIES
Azotemia
Increased alanine aminotransferase (ALT) activity
Increased aspartate aminotransferase activity
Increased lactate dehydrogenase activity
Increased creatine kinase activity
Hyperglycemia
Lymphopenia
Disseminated intravascular coagulation (DIC)

## Aspiration Pneumonia

### Etiology of Aspiration Pneumonia

#### ESOPHAGEAL DISORDERS
Megaesophagus
Reflux esophagitis
Esophageal obstruction
Myasthenia gravis (localized)
Bronchoesophageal fistulae

#### LOCALIZED OROPHARYNGEAL DISORDERS
Cleft palate
Cricopharyngeal motor dysfunction
Brachycephalic airway syndrome
Laryngeal paralysis

#### SYSTEMIC NEUROMUSCULAR DISORDERS
Myasthenia gravis
Polyneuropathy
Polymyopathy

#### DECREASED MENTATION
General anesthesia
Sedation
Post ictus

Head trauma
Severe metabolic disease

## IATROGENIC
Force feeding
Stomach tubes

## VOMITING (IN COMBINATION WITH OTHER PREDISPOSING FACTORS)

# Atrioventricular Valve Disease, Chronic (Mitral or Tricuspid Valve)

## Potential Complications

### ACUTE WORSENING OF PULMONARY EDEMA
Arrhythmias
    Frequent atrial premature contractions
    Paroxysmal atrial/supraventricular contractions
    Atrial fibrillation
    Ventricular tachyarrhythmias
    Rule out drug toxicity (e.g., digoxin)
Ruptured chordae tendineae
Iatrogenic volume overload
    Excessive fluid or blood administration
    High-sodium fluids
High-sodium intake
Increased cardiac workload
    Physical exertion
    Anemia
    Infection/sepsis
    Hypertension
Disease of other organ systems (pulmonary, hepatic, renal, endocrine)
    Environmental stress (heat, humidity, cold, etc.)
    Inadequate medication for stage of disease
Erratic or improper drug administration
Myocardial degeneration and poor contractility

### CAUSES OF REDUCED CARDIAC OUTPUT
Arrhythmias
Ruptured chordae tendineae
Cough-related syncope
Left atrial tear, intrapericardial bleeding, cardiac tamponade
Secondary right-sided heart failure
Myocardial degeneration, poor contractility
Increased cardiac workload

## Canine Infectious Tracheobronchitis, Etiologic Agents Associated With

Usually a multietiologic disease involving one or more of the following:

- *Bordetella bronchiseptica*
- Canine parainfluenza virus
- Canine adenovirus 2
- Canine influenza virus
- Canine herpesvirus
- Canine respiratory coronavirus
- *Mycoplasma* spp.
- *Streptococcus equi* subsp. *zooepidemicus*
- Canine distemper virus

Most frequent combination is *B. bronchiseptica* with canine parainfluenza virus or canine adenovirus

## Cardiomegaly

### Differential Diagnosis

#### GENERALIZED CARDIOMEGALY
Dilated cardiomyopathy
Pericardial effusion (radiographic image looks like generalized cardiomegaly)
Mitral and tricuspid valve insufficiency
Tricuspid dysplasia
Pericardioperitoneal diaphragmatic hernia
Ventricular septal defect
Patent ductus arteriosus

#### LEFT ATRIAL ENLARGEMENT
Mitral valve insufficiency
Hypertrophic cardiomyopathy
Early dilated cardiomyopathy (especially in Doberman Pinschers)
Subaortic or aortic stenosis

#### LEFT ATRIAL AND VENTRICULAR ENLARGEMENT
Dilated cardiomyopathy
Hypertrophic cardiomyopathy
Mitral valve insufficiency
Aortic valve insufficiency
Ventricular septal defect
Patent ductus arteriosus
Subaortic or aortic stenosis
Systemic hypertension
Hyperthyroidism

### RIGHT ATRIAL AND VENTRICULAR ENLARGEMENT

Advanced heartworm disease
Chronic severe pulmonary disease
Tricuspid valve insufficiency
Atrial septal defect
Pulmonic stenosis
Tetralogy of Fallot
Reverse-shunting congenital defects
Pulmonary hypertension
Mass lesion within right heart

## Chylothorax

### Diagnostic Criteria

Protein concentration is greater than 2.5 g/dL
Nucleated cell count ranges from 400–10,000/mL
Predominant cell type on cytology is the small lymphocyte
(also see neutrophils, macrophages, plasma cells, and
mesothelial cells)
Triglyceride concentration of pleural fluid is greater than
that of serum (definitive test)

### Diagnostic Tests to Identify Underlying Disease

Cytologic examination of fluid
- Neoplastic cells
- Infectious agents

Thoracic radiography (after fluid removal)
- Cranial mediastinal masses
- Other neoplasia
- Cardiac disease
- Heartworm disease
- Pericardial disease

Ultrasonography (in the presence of fluid)
- Cranial mediastinum
- Mass
- Echocardiography
- Cardiomyopathy
- Heartworm disease
- Pericardial disease
- Congenital heart disease

Ultrasound of fluid pockets near body wall
- Neoplasia
- Lung lobe torsion

Laboratory tests
- Heartworm antibody and antigen tests
- Complete blood count (CBC)

- Serum biochemical profile
- Urinalysis

Lymphangiography

- Preoperative and postoperative assessment of thoracic duct

Computed tomography

## Causes of Chylothorax

### TRAUMATIC

Blunt force trauma (e.g., vehicular trauma)

Postthoracotomy

### NONTRAUMATIC

Neoplasia (especially mediastinal lymphoma in cats)

Cardiomyopathy

Dirofilariasis

Pericardial disease

Other causes of right heart failure

Lung lobe torsion

Diaphragmatic hernia

Systemic lymphangiectasia

Cranial vena cava thrombosis (may be associated with implantation of a device like a pacemaker lead in the jugular vein)

### IDIOPATHIC (MOST COMMONLY DIAGNOSED)

## Diagnostic Tests to Identify Underlying Cause of Chylothorax in Dogs and Cats

### CBC, SERUM CHEMISTRY, URINALYSIS

Evaluation of systemic status

### CYTOLOGIC EXAMINATION OF PLEURAL FLUID

Infectious agents

Neoplastic cells

### THORACIC RADIOGRAPHS (AFTER FLUID REMOVAL)

Cranial mediastinal masses

Other neoplasia

Cardiac disease

Heartworm disease

Pericardial disease

### ULTRASONOGRAPHY (BEFORE FLUID REMOVAL)

Cranial mediastinum (masses)

Echocardiography (cardiomyopathy, heartworm disease, pericardial disease, congenital heart disease)

Ultrasound of body wall and pleural space (neoplasia, lung lobe torsion)

### HEARTWORM ANTIBODY AND ANTIGEN TESTS
Heartworm disease

### LYMPHANGIOGRAPHY
Preoperative and postoperative assessment of thoracic duct

## Congenital Heart Disease

### Breed Predispositions

#### PATENT DUCTUS ARTERIOSUS
Maltese, Pomeranian, Shetland Sheepdog, English Cocker Spaniel, English Springer Spaniel, Keeshond, Bichon Frise, Toy and Miniature Poodle, Yorkshire Terrier, Collie, Cocker Spaniel, Corgi, German Shepherd, Chihuahua, Kerry Blue Terrier, Labrador Retriever, Newfoundland; females affected more than males

#### SUBAORTIC STENOSIS
Newfoundland, Golden Retriever, Rottweiler, Boxer, German Shepherd, English Bulldog, Great Dane, German Shorthaired Pointer, Bouvier des Flandres, Samoyed

#### AORTIC STENOSIS
Bull Terrier

#### PULMONIC STENOSIS
English Bulldog (males affected more than females), Mastiff, Samoyed, Miniature Schnauzer, Newfoundland, West Highland White Terrier, Cocker Spaniel, Beagle, Basset Hound, Airedale Terrier, Boykin Spaniel, Chihuahua, Scottish Terrier, Boxer, Fox Terrier, Chow Chow, Labrador Retriever, Schnauzer, Miniature Pinscher

#### ATRIAL SEPTAL DEFECT
Samoyed, Doberman Pinscher, Boxer

#### VENTRICULAR SEPTAL DEFECT
English Bulldog, English Springer Spaniel, Keeshond, West Highland White Terrier, cats

#### TRICUSPID DYSPLASIA
Labrador Retriever, German Shepherd, Boxer, Weimaraner, Great Dane, Old English Sheepdog, Golden Retriever, various other large breeds

### MITRAL DYSPLASIA
Bull Terrier, German Shepherd, Great Dane, Golden
Retriever, Newfoundland, Dalmatian, Mastiff,
Rottweiler, cats

### TETRALOGY OF FALLOT
Keeshond, English Bulldog

### PERSISTENT RIGHT AORTIC ARCH
German Shepherd, Great Dane, Irish Setter

### COR TRIATRIATUM
Medium- to large-breed dogs (Chow Chow), rarely small-
breed dogs or cats

### PERITONEOPERICARDIAL DIAPHRAGMATIC HERNIA
Weimaraner

## Heart Failure

### Causes of Chronic Heart Failure

#### LEFT-SIDED HEART FAILURE
*Volume-Flow Overload*
Mitral valve regurgitation (degenerative, congenital,
infective)
Aortic regurgitation (infective endocardiosis,
congenital)
Ventricular septal defect
Patent ductus arteriosus

*Myocardial Failure*
Myocardial ischemia/infarction
Drug toxicity (e.g., doxorubicin)

*Pressure Overload*
Aortic/subaortic stenosis
Systemic hypertension

*Restriction of Ventricular Filling*
Hypertrophic cardiomyopathy
Restrictive cardiomyopathy

#### LEFT- OR RIGHT-SIDED HEART FAILURE
*Myocardial Failure*
Idiopathic dilated cardiomyopathy
Infective myocarditis

*Volume-Flow Overload*
Chronic anemia
Thyrotoxicosis

## RIGHT-SIDED HEART FAILURE

### Volume-Flow Overload
Tricuspid endocarditis
Tricuspid endocardiosis
Tricuspid dysplasia

### Pressure Overload
Pulmonic stenosis
Heartworm disease
Pulmonary hypertension

### Restriction to Ventricular Filling
Cardiac tamponade
Constrictive pericardial disease

### Sustained Tachyarrhythmias
Supraventricular tachycardia
Atrial fibrillation

### Chronic Bradyarrhythmias
Complete heart block

## Severity

### CLASSIFICATION SYSTEMS

#### New York Heart Association Functional Classification
**Class I:** Heart disease present but no evidence of heart failure or exercise intolerance; cardiomegaly minimal to absent

**Class II:** Signs of heart disease with evidence of exercise intolerance; radiographic cardiomegaly present

**Class III:** Signs of heart failure with normal activity or signs at night (e.g., cough, orthopnea); radiographic signs of significant cardiomegaly and pulmonary edema or pleural/abdominal effusion

**Class IV:** Severe heart failure with clinical signs at rest or with minimal activity; marked radiographic signs of congestive heart failure (CHF) and cardiomegaly

#### International Small Animal Cardiac Health Council Functional Classification
**Class I:** Asymptomatic patient

**Class Ia:** Signs of heart disease without cardiomegaly

**Class Ib:** Signs of heart disease and evidence of compensation (cardiomegaly)

**Class II:** Mild to moderate heart failure; clinical signs of failure evident at rest or with mild exercise and adversely affect quality of life

**Class III:** Advanced heart failure; clinical signs of CHF are immediately obvious

**Class IIIa:** Home care is possible

**Class IIIb:** Hospitalization recommended (cardiogenic shock, life-threatening edema, large pleural effusion, refractory ascites)

## Clinical Findings

### LOW-OUTPUT SIGNS

Exercise intolerance
Syncope
Weak arterial pulses
Tachycardia
Arrhythmias
Cold extremities
Prerenal azotemia
Cyanosis

### SIGNS RELATED TO POOR SKELETAL MUSCLE FUNCTION

Weight loss
Exercise intolerance
Dyspnea
Decreased muscle mass

### SIGNS RELATED TO FLUID RETENTION

*Left-Sided Heart Failure (Pulmonary Edema)*

Dyspnea/orthopnea
Exercise intolerance
Wet lung sounds
Tachypnea
Gallop rhythm
Functional mitral regurgitation
Cyanosis
Cough

*Right-Sided Heart Failure*

Ascites
Subcutaneous edema
Jugular distension/pulsation
Hepatomegaly
Splenomegaly
Hepatojugular reflux
Gallop rhythm
Cardiac arrhythmias
Pleural effusion
Pericardial effusion (small)

*Bilateral Signs*

Pleural effusion (dyspnea, muffled heart sounds, cough)

## Heartworm Disease

### Clinical Findings

#### HISTORICAL FINDINGS
Asymptomatic
Cough
Dyspnea
Weight loss
Lethargy
Exercise intolerance
Poor condition
Syncope
Abdominal distension (ascites)

#### PHYSICAL FINDINGS
Weight loss
Right-sided murmur (tricuspid insufficiency)
Split-second heart sound
Gallop rhythm
Cough
Pulmonary crackles
Dyspnea
Muffled breath sounds
Cyanosis
Right-sided heart failure
- Jugular distension/pulsation
- Hepatosplenomegaly
- Ascites
Pulmonary thromboembolism
- Dyspnea/tachypnea
- Fever
- Hemoptysis
Cardiac arrhythmias/conduction disturbances (rare)
Caval syndrome
- Hemoglobinuria
- Anemia
- DIC
- Icterus
- Collapse/death

#### CLINICOPATHOLOGIC FINDINGS
Eosinophilia
Nonregenerative anemia
Neutrophilia
Basophilia
Monocytosis
Polyclonal gammopathy

Proteinuria
Hyperbilirubinemia
Azotemia
Thrombocytopenia
Mild to moderate hepatic enzyme elevation

## RADIOGRAPHIC SIGNS

Right ventricular enlargement
Prominent main pulmonary artery segment
Increased pulmonary artery size
Tortuous pulmonary vessels
Caudal vena cava enlargement
Hepatosplenomegaly
Ascites
Pleural effusion
Bronchial/interstitial lung disease

## ECHOCARDIOGRAPHY

Caudal vena cava distension
Right ventricular hypertrophy
Ascites
Pleural effusion
Pericardial effusion
Tricuspid regurgitation demonstrated by color-flow
   Doppler imaging
Worms seen as small, bright parallel echoes within pul-
   monary artery, right ventricle, right atrium, vena cava

## DIAGNOSIS IN DOGS

*Antigen Test Positive and Modified Knott or Filter
Test Negative*
   Perform CBC, serum chemistry panel, urinalysis,
      thoracic radiography

*Antigen Test Positive and Modified Knott or Filter
Test Positive*
   Perform CBC, serum chemistry panel, urinalysis,
      thoracic radiography

*Antigen Test Negative*
   No infection or low heartworm burden
   Start preventative

## CLASSIFICATION OF HEARTWORM DISEASE SEVERITY IN DOGS

*Class 1 (Mild)*
   No clinical signs or occasional cough, fatigue with
      exercise, mild loss of condition
   No radiographic or clinicopathologic abnormalities

*Class 2 (Moderate)*

No clinical signs or occasional cough, fatigue with exercise, mild to moderate loss of condition

Radiographic evidence of right ventricular enlargement, mild pulmonary arterial enlargement, perivascular and/or mixed alveolar/interstitial opacities

± Mild anemia

*Class 3 (Severe)*

General loss of condition/cachexia, fatigue with exercise, persistent cough ± dyspnea ± right-sided heart failure

Radiography shows right ventricular enlargement ± right atrial enlargement, moderate to severe pulmonary artery enlargement, perivascular or diffuse mixed alveolar/interstitial opacities ± evidence of thromboembolism

Anemia, proteinuria

*Class 4 (Caval Syndrome)*

Acute onset of lethargy, dyspnea, pallor, weakness, collapse, and death.

Radiographic signs are similar to class 3.

## Hypertension

### Pulmonary Hypertension

#### POTENTIAL CLINICAL SIGNS

Ascites

Jugular venous distension/pulsation

Subcutaneous edema

Cachexia

Exercise intolerance, weakness

Syncope

Nonspecific respiratory signs
- Coughing
- Tachypnea
- Respiratory distress
- Increased bronchovesicular sounds
- Hemoptysis

Cyanosis
- Right-to-left cardiac shunts
- Severe respiratory disease

Split or loud pulmonic component to second heart sound

Right or left apical systolic murmurs (tricuspid or mitral regurgitation)

## RADIOGRAPHIC SIGNS
Cardiomegaly
Right ventricular enlargement
Dilated central pulmonary arteries with tapering toward periphery
Eisenmenger complex (pulmonary undercirculation and right-sided heart enlargement)
Left atrial enlargement and perihilar to caudodorsal pulmonary infiltrates (left-sided CHF)

## ECHOCARDIOGRAPHIC SIGNS
Right ventricular concentric hypertrophy and dilation
Main pulmonary artery and main branch dilation
Systolic flattening of interventricular septum
Paradoxical septal motion
Reduced left ventricular dimensions in severe pulmonary hypertension caused by ventricular underfilling
Vena cava distension

## LABORATORY VALUES
Acidosis
Rule out heartworm disease

# Systemic Hypertension

## CAUSES OF SYSTEMIC HYPERTENSION IN DOGS AND CATS
Renal failure (chronic or acute)
Hyperadrenocorticism
Diabetes mellitus
Pheochromocytoma
Hyperthyroidism
Liver disease
Hyperaldosteronism
Intracranial lesions (intracranial pressure)
High-salt diet
Obesity
Chronic anemia (cats)

## CLINICAL SIGNS OF SYSTEMIC HYPERTENSION
### Ocular Findings
Hypertensive choroidopathy (edema, vascular tortuosity, hemorrhage, focal ischemia)
Hypertensive retinopathy (edema, vascular tortuosity, hemorrhage, focal ischemia, atrophy)
Intraocular hemorrhage (retinal, vitreal, hyphema)
Retinal detachment
Papilledema
Blindness
Glaucoma
Secondary corneal ulcers

*Neurologic Findings*
  Edema (intracranial pressure)
  Hypertensive encephalopathy (lethargy, behavioral changes)
  Cerebrovascular accident (focal ischemia, hemorrhage)
  Seizures/collapse
  Vestibular signs

*Renal*
  Polyuria/polydipsia
  Glomerulosclerosis/proliferative glomerulitis
  Renal tubular degeneration and fibrosis
  Further deterioration in renal function
  Proteinuria

*Cardiac*
  Left ventricular hypertrophy
  Murmur or gallop sound
  Aortic dilation
  Aneurysm or dissection (rare)
  Left-sided CHF (rare)

*Other*
  Epistaxis

## Laryngeal and Pharyngeal Disease

## Differential Diagnosis

Laryngeal paralysis
Brachycephalic airway syndrome
Acute laryngitis
Laryngeal neoplasia
Nasopharyngeal polyp
Abscess
Tonsillitis
Pharyngitis
Obstructive laryngitis
Laryngeal collapse
Trauma
Foreign body
Extraluminal mass
Elongated soft palate
Cleft palate
Soft palate hypoplasia
Pharyngeal neoplasia
Granuloma
Pharyngeal mucoceles

Web formation
Nasopharyngeal stenosis

## Causes of Laryngeal Paralysis

### IDIOPATHIC

### POLYNEUROPATHY AND POLYMYOPATHY

Idiopathic
Immune-mediated
Endocrinopathy
- Hypothyroidism
- Hypoadrenocorticism

Toxicity
Congenital disease

### VENTRAL CERVICAL LESION

Nerve trauma
- Direct trauma
- Inflammation
- Fibrosis

Neoplasia
Other inflammatory or mass lesion

### ANTERIOR THORACIC LESION

Neoplasia
Trauma
- Postoperative
- Other

Other inflammatory or mass lesion

### MYASTHENIA GRAVIS

## Lower Respiratory Tract Disease

## Differential Diagnosis

### DISORDERS OF TRACHEA AND BRONCHI

Canine infectious tracheobronchitis
Collapsing trachea
Bacterial infection
Mycoplasmal infection
Bronchial asthma
Neoplasia
Allergic bronchitis
Feline bronchitis
Bronchial compression
- Left atrial enlargement
- Hilar lymphadenopathy

Acute bronchitis
Canine chronic bronchitis/bronchiectasis

Parasites (*Oslerus osleri, Filaroides osleri*)
Tracheal tear/avulsion
Primary ciliary dyskinesia
Airway foreign body
Chronic aspiration

## DISORDERS OF PULMONARY PARENCHYMA

Infectious disease
- Viral pneumonia (canine influenza, canine distemper virus, canine adenovirus, canine parainfluenza, feline calicivirus, feline infectious peritonitis [FIP], pneumonia secondary to feline leukemia virus [FeLV] or feline immunodeficiency virus [FIV])
- Bacterial pneumonia
- Protozoal pneumonia (toxoplasmosis)
- Fungal pneumonia (blastomycosis, histoplasmosis, coccidioidomycosis)
- Rickettsial disease (*Rickettsia rickettsii, Ehrlichia* spp.)
- Parasitism
- Heartworm disease
- Pulmonary parasites (*Paragonimus, Aelurostrongylus, Capillaria, Crenosoma* spp.)
- Larval migration of *Toxocara canis*

Aspiration pneumonia
Pulmonary infiltrates with eosinophils
Eosinophilic pulmonary granulomatosis
Pulmonary neoplasia (primary, metastatic, lympho-sarcoma, lymphomatoid granulomatosis, malignant histiocytosis)
Pulmonary hypertension
Pulmonary contusions
Pulmonary thromboembolism
Pulmonary edema
Acute respiratory distress syndrome (ARDS)
Lung lobe torsion
Pulmonary fibrosis
Pickwickian syndrome (obesity)
Idiopathic interstitial pneumonias

## Mediastinal Disease

### Differential Diagnosis of Lesions Associated With Focal Mediastinal Enlargement

Pneumomediastinum
Mediastinitis (*Histoplasma, Cryptococcus, Actinomyces, Nocardia, Spirocerca* spp.)

Mediastinal hemorrhage
Mediastinal cysts
Nonneoplastic mediastinal masses (fungal pyogranulomas, abscesses, granulomas, lymphadenopathy, hematomas)
Mediastinal neoplasia (lymphosarcoma)
Thymoma
Obesity
Thymic hemorrhage
Heart base mass
Neurogenic tumor
Tracheal mass
Esophageal mass, foreign body, or dilatation
Ectopic thyroid tissue
Mediastinal edema
Vascular mass (aorta, cranial vena cava)
Paraspinal or spinal mass
Aortic stenosis
Patent ductus arteriosus
Left atrial enlargement
Main pulmonary artery mass (poststenotic dilatation)
Hiatal hernia
Diaphragmatic hernia or mass
Aortic aneurysm
Gastroesophageal intussusception
Peritoneopericardial diaphragmatic hernia

## Murmurs

### Clinical Findings

#### SYSTOLIC MURMURS

Functional murmurs (point of maximal impulse [PMI] over left-sided heart base, decrescendo or crescendo–decrescendo)
- Innocent puppy murmurs
- Physiologic murmurs (anemia, fever, high sympathetic tone, hyperthyroidism, peripheral arteriovenous fistula, marked bradycardia, hypoproteinemia, athletic heart)

Mitral valve insufficiency (left apex, typically holosystolic)
Ejection murmurs (typically left-sided heart base)
- Subaortic stenosis (low left base and right base)
- Pulmonic stenosis (high left base)
- Dynamic muscular obstruction

Right-sided murmurs (usually holosystolic)
- Tricuspid insufficiency (right apex, may see jugular pulse)
- Ventricular septal defect (PMI over right sternal border)

### DIASTOLIC MURMURS

Aortic insufficiency from bacterial endocarditis (left-sided heart base)

Aortic valve congenital malformations (left base)

Aortic valve degenerative disease (left base)

Pulmonic insufficiency (left base)

### CONTINUOUS MURMURS

Patent ductus arteriosus (PMI high left base above pulmonic area)

### CONCURRENT SYSTOLIC AND DIASTOLIC MURMURS (TO-AND-FRO MURMURS)

Subaortic stenosis with aortic insufficiency

Ventricular septal defect and aortic insufficiency

Pulmonic stenosis with pulmonic insufficiency

## Grading

**Grade I:** Very soft murmur; heard only in quiet surroundings after minutes of listening

**Grade II:** Soft murmur but easily heard

**Grade III:** Moderate-intensity murmur

**Grade IV:** Loud murmur; no precordial thrill

**Grade V:** Loud murmur with palpable precordial thrill

**Grade VI:** Very loud murmur; can be heard with stethoscope off chest wall; palpable precordial thrill

## Myocardial Diseases

## Differential Diagnosis, Dogs

### DILATED CARDIOMYOPATHY

*Primary (Idiopathic, Most Common)*

Genetic (Doberman Pinscher, Boxer, Cocker Spaniel, Great Dane, Portuguese Water Dog, Newfoundland, Dalmatian, Irish Wolfhound, Old English Sheepdog, Scottish Deerhound; Abyssinian, Burmese, and Siamese cats overrepresented)

*Secondary*

Nutritional Deficiencies

L-Carnitine (Boxer, Doberman Pinscher, Great Dane, Irish Wolfhound, Newfoundland, Cocker Spaniel)

Taurine

Grain-free diet–related myocardial failure

Myocardial Infection
- Viral myocarditis (acute viral infections, e.g., parvovirus, West Nile virus)
- Bacterial myocarditis (secondary to bacteremia from infections elsewhere in body)
- Bartonellosis
- Lyme disease: *Borrelia burgdorferi*
- Protozoal myocarditis (*Trypanosoma cruzi* [Chagas disease], *Toxoplasma gondii, Neospora caninum, Babesia canis, Hepatozoon canis*)
- Fungal myocarditis (rare, *Aspergillus, Cryptococcus, Coccidioides, Histoplasma, Paecilomyces* spp.)
- Rickettsial myocarditis (rare, *Rickettsia rickettsii, Ehrlichia canis, Bartonella* spp.),
- Algaelike organisms (rare, *Prototheca* spp.)
- Nematode larval migration (*Toxocara* spp.)

Trauma
- Hit by car
- Blunt trauma from falling
- Penetrating trauma
- Cardiac catheterization

Ischemia

Infiltrative Neoplasia

Hyperthermia

Irradiation

Electric Shock

Cardiotoxins
- Doxorubicin; ethyl alcohol; plant toxins such as foxglove, black locust, buttercup, lily of the valley, and gossypol; cocaine; anesthetic drugs; catecholamines; monensin
- Transmissible myocarditis–diaphragmitis of cats

## HYPERTROPHIC CARDIOMYOPATHY (UNCOMMON IN DOGS)

## ARRHYTHMOGENIC RIGHT VENTRICULAR CARDIOMYOPATHY (RARE)

## NONINFECTIVE MYOCARDITIS

Catecholamines; heavy metals; antineoplastic drugs (doxorubicin, cyclophosphamide, 5-fluorouracil, interleukin-2, interferon-α); stimulant drugs (thyroid hormone, cocaine, amphetamines, lithium)

Immune-mediated diseases, pheochromocytoma

Wasp and scorpion stings, snake venom, spider bite

## Differential Diagnosis, Cats

### HYPERTROPHIC CARDIOMYOPATHY

*Primary (Idiopathic)*
> Maine Coon, Persian, Ragdoll, and American Shorthair may be predisposed.

*Secondary*
> Hyperthyroidism
> Hypersomatotropism (acromegaly)
> Infiltrative myocardial disease (lymphoma)

### RESTRICTIVE CARDIOMYOPATHY

### DILATED CARDIOMYOPATHY
Taurine-deficient diets
Doxorubicin
End-stage of other myocardial metabolic, toxic, or infectious process

### ARRHYTHMOGENIC RIGHT VENTRICULAR CARDIOMYOPATHY

### MYOCARDITIS
Viral (coronavirus, other viruses)
Bacterial (bacteremia, *Bartonella* spp.)
Protozoal (*Toxoplasma gondii*)

## Pericardial Effusion

## Differential Diagnosis

### BACTERIAL PERICARDITIS
Secondary to foxtail (*Hordeum* spp.) migration
Secondary to penetrating animal bite
Disseminated tuberculosis

### FUNGAL PERICARDITIS
Coccidioidomycosis
Aspergillosis
Actinomycosis

### VIRAL PERICARDITIS
FIP
Canine distemper virus

### PROTOZOAL PERICARDITIS
Toxoplasmosis
Other systemic protozoal infections

## LEFT ATRIAL RUPTURE (SECONDARY TO MITRAL VALVE DISEASE)

## NEOPLASIA
Hemangiosarcoma
Mesothelioma
Heart base tumor (aortic body tumor, chemodectoma, ectopic thyroid tumor, ectopic parathyroid tumor, connective tissue neoplasms)
Fibrosarcoma
Lymphosarcoma
Rhabdomyosarcoma

## OTHER
Penetrating trauma
Pericardioperitoneal diaphragmatic hernia
Hypoalbuminemia
Pericardial cyst
Coagulation disorders
CHF
Uremia
Idiopathic

# Pleural Effusion

## Differential Diagnosis

### TRANSUDATES AND MODIFIED TRANSUDATES
Right-sided heart failure
Pericardial disease
Hypoalbuminemia
Neoplasia
Diaphragmatic hernia

### NONSEPTIC EXUDATES
FIP
Neoplasia
Diaphragmatic hernia
Lung lobe torsion

### SEPTIC EXUDATES
Pyothorax

### CHYLOUS EFFUSION
Chylothorax

### HEMORRHAGE
Trauma
Bleeding disorder
Neoplasia
Lung lobe torsion

## Diagnostic Approach in Dogs and Cats With Pleural Effusion Based on Fluid Type

### PURE AND MODIFIED TRANSUDATES

Right-sided heart failure, pericardial effusion (evaluate pulses, auscultation, electrocardiogram [ECG], thoracic radiography, echocardiography)

Hypoalbuminemia (serum albumin concentration)

Neoplasia, diaphragmatic hernia (thoracic radiography, thoracic ultrasound, computed tomography [CT], thoracoscopy, thoracotomy)

### NONSEPTIC EXUDATES

FIP (pleural fluid cytology [most reliable test], CBC, serum chemistry, ophthalmoscopic examination, serum or fluid electrophoresis, coronavirus antibody titer, polymerase chain reaction [PCR] of tissues or effusion)

Neoplasia, diaphragmatic hernia (thoracic radiography, thoracic ultrasound, CT, thoracoscopy, thoracotomy)

Lung lobe torsion (thoracic radiography, ultrasound, bronchoscopy, thoracotomy)

### SEPTIC EXUDATES

Pyothorax (Gram stain, aerobic and anaerobic culture, cytology)

### CHYLOUS EFFUSION

Chylothorax (protein concentration, nucleated cell count, cytology, triglyceride)

### HEMORRHAGIC

Trauma (history)

Bleeding disorder (systemic examination, coagulation tests, platelet count)

Neoplasia (thoracic radiography, thoracic ultrasound, CT, thoracoscopy, thoracotomy)

Lung lobe torsion (thoracic radiography, ultrasound, bronchoscopy, thoracotomy)

## Pulmonary Disease

## Differential Diagnosis Based on Radiographic Patterns

### ALVEOLAR PATTERN

Pulmonary edema (cardiogenic or noncardiogenic)

Infectious pneumonia (bacterial, parasitic, protozoal, viral)

Aspiration pneumonia

Atelectasis
Drowning
Smoke inhalation
ARDS
Hemorrhage
- Neoplasia (primary and metastatic)
- Fungal pneumonia (severe)
- Pulmonary contusion
- Thromboembolic disease
- Systemic coagulopathy

## BRONCHIAL PATTERN

Feline bronchitis/asthma
Allergic bronchitis
Bacterial bronchitis
Canine chronic bronchitis
Bronchiectasis
Pulmonary parasites
Bronchial calcification

## VASCULAR PATTERN

*Enlarged Arteries*
Heartworm disease
Thromboembolic disease
Pulmonary hypertension

*Enlarged Veins*
Left-sided heart failure

*Enlarged Arteries and Veins (Pulmonary
Overcirculation)*

*Left-to-Right Shunts*
Patent ductus arteriosus
Ventricular septal defect
Atrial septal defect

*Small Arteries and Veins*
Pulmonary Undercirculation
Cardiovascular shock
Hypovolemia
- Severe dehydration
- Blood loss
- Hypoadrenocorticism
Pulmonic valve stenosis

Hyperinflation of Lungs
Feline bronchitis
Allergic bronchitis

## NODULAR INTERSTITIAL PATTERN

Mycotic infection
- Blastomycosis
- Histoplasmosis
- Coccidioidomycosis

Neoplasia

Pulmonary parasites
- *Aelurostrongylus* infection
- *Paragonimus* infection
- Pulmonary abscess
- Bacterial pneumonia
- Foreign body

Pulmonary infiltrates with eosinophils
Miscellaneous inflammatory diseases
Inactive lesions

## RETICULAR INTERSTITIAL PATTERNS

Infection
- Viral pneumonia
- Bacterial pneumonia
- Toxoplasmosis
- Mycotic pneumonia

Parasitic infestation
Neoplasia
Pulmonary fibrosis
Eosinophilic lung disease
Miscellaneous inflammatory diseases
Hemorrhage (mild)
Old dog lung

## Pulmonary Edema

### Causes

#### VASCULAR OVERLOAD

Cardiogenic
- Left-sided heart murmur
- Left-to-right shunt

Overhydration

#### DECREASED PLASMA ONCOTIC PRESSURE

Hypoalbuminemia
- Gastrointestinal (GI) loss
- Renal loss (glomerular disease)
- Liver disease (lack of production)
- Iatrogenic overhydration
- Starvation

## INCREASED VASCULAR PERMEABILITY

Sepsis or systemic inflammatory response (SIRS)

Shock

Drugs or toxins

Snake envenomation

Cisplatin (cats)

Trauma

- Pulmonary
- Multisystemic

Inhaled toxins

- Smoke inhalation
- Gastric acid aspiration
- Oxygen toxicity

Electrocution

Pancreatitis

Uremia

Virulent babesiosis

DIC

Inflammation/vasculitis

## OTHER CAUSES

Thromboembolism

Postobstruction (strangulation, laryngeal paralysis, pulmonary reexpansion)

Near-drowning

Neurogenic edema

- Seizures
- Head trauma

Lung lobe torsion

Bacterial pneumonia

Pulmonary contusion

Hyperoxia

High altitude

Air embolus

Pheochromocytoma

## LYMPHATIC OBSTRUCTION (RARE)

Neoplasia

## Pulmonary Thromboembolism

### Causes

#### EMBOLIZATION OF THROMBI (ANY CONDITION THAT PREDISPOSES TO VENOUS STASIS, ENDOTHELIAL INJURY, AND HYPERCOAGULABILITY)

Heartworm disease

Immune-mediated hemolytic anemia

Systemic inflammatory disease
Neoplasia
Cardiac disease
Cardiomyopathy
Endocarditis
CHF
Protein-losing nephropathy
Protein-losing enteropathy
Hyperadrenocorticism
Pancreatitis
DIC
Anatomic abnormality (e.g., aneurysm, AV fistula)
Hyperviscosity (polycythemia, leukemia, hyperglobulinemia)
Hypoviscosity (anemia)
Sepsis
Shock
Intravenous catheterization
Injection of irritating substance
Prolonged recumbency
Reperfusion injury
Atherosclerosis/arteriosclerosis
Trauma
Recent surgery
Hyperhomocysteinemia
Vasculitis

**EMBOLIZATION OF PARASITES**
Heartworm disease

**EMBOLIZATION OF FAT**

**EMBOLIZATION OF NEOPLASTIC CELLS**

## Tachycardia, Sinus

### Causes

Anxiety/fear
Excitement
Exercise
Pain
Hyperthyroidism
Hyperthermia/fever
Anemia
CHF
Hypoxia

Shock
Hypotension
Sepsis
Drugs (anticholinergics, sympathomimetics)
Toxicity (e.g., chocolate, hexachlorophene)
Electric shock

# Dermatologic Disorders

## Allergic Skin Disease

### Clinical Findings

#### FLEA ALLERGY

*Dogs*

Papular rash
Caudal distribution of lesions most common

*Cats*

Miliary dermatitis, especially over caudal back, around neck and chin
Eosinophilic granuloma complex

#### ATOPY AND CUTANEOUS SIGNS OF FOOD HYPERSENSITIVITY

Signs of these two types of allergies are similar.

Atopy tends to occur primarily in young adults, whereas food hypersensitivity can begin at any age. Atopy is usually seasonal at first but may become less seasonal.

*Dogs*

Papular rash
Pruritus and self-trauma
Lesions of face, ears, feet, and perineum
Recurrent otitis externa
Excoriation
Lichenification
Pigmentary changes
Secondary pyoderma

*Cats*

Miliary dermatitis
Eosinophilic dermatitis

## ALLERGIC CONTACT DERMATITIS
Rarest of allergic dermatoses
Lesions tend to be confined to hairless or sparsely
haired skin (ventral abdomen, neck, and chest;
ventral paws but not pads; perineum; lateral aspect of
pinnae)
Acutely: erythema, macules, papules, vesicles
Chronically: alopecic plaques, hyperpigmentation,
hypopigmentation, excoriation, lichenification

## Alopecia, Endocrine
### Causes
Hypothyroidism
Hyperadrenocorticism
Diabetes mellitus
Adrenal sex hormone deficiency (alopecia X)
Growth hormone deficiency (pituitary dwarfism)
Growth hormone–responsive dermatosis in adult dogs
Castration-responsive dermatosis
Hyperestrogenism
• Sertoli cell tumor (male dog)
• Intact female dog
Hypoestrogenism (poorly understood)
• Estrogen-responsive dermatosis of spayed female dogs
• Feline endocrine alopecia
Hypoandrogenism
• Testosterone-responsive dermatosis (male dog)
• Feline endocrine alopecia
Telogen defluxion (effluvium): often after recent pregnancy
or diestrus
Progestin excess (excess of progesterone or
17-hydroxyprogesterone)

### Clinical Findings
#### NONSPECIFIC FEATURES OF ENDOCRINE DISEASE
Bilaterally symmetric alopecia
Follicular dilation, follicular keratosis, follicular atrophy
Orthokeratotic hyperkeratosis
Predominance of telogen hair follicles
Sebaceous gland atrophy
Epidermal atrophy
Thin dermis
Epidermal melanosis
Dermal collagen atrophy

**FEATURES SUGGESTIVE OF SPECIFIC ENDOCRINE DISORDER**

Hypothyroidism
- Vacuolated and/or hypertrophied arrector pili muscles, increased dermal mucin content, thick dermis

Hyperadrenocorticism
- Calcinosis cutis, comedones, absence of erector pili muscles

Hyposomatotropism
- Decreased amount and size of dermal elastin fibers

Growth-hormone– and castration-responsive dermatoses
- Excessive trichilemmal keratinization (flame follicles)

## Claw Disorders

### Definitions

Onychodystrophy: claw malformation

Onychogryphosis: hypertrophic claw with abnormal curvature

Onycholysis: separation of claw from underlying corium

Onychomadesis: sloughing of claw

Onychomycosis: fungal infection of claw

Onychorrhexis: brittle claws that tend to split or break

Paronychia: inflammation of soft tissue around claw

Symmetric lupoid onychodystrophy/onychitis (SLO):lupus-like disorder that cause onychomadesis and subsequent onychodystrophy of multiple claws

### Differential Diagnosis for Abnormal Claws

**BACTERIAL CLAW INFECTION—ALMOST ALWAYS SECONDARY TO AN UNDERLYING CAUSE**

Trauma—usually one claw affected

Hypothyroidism

Hyperadrenocorticism

Diabetes mellitus

Allergies

Autoimmune disorders

Symmetrical lupoid onychodystrophy

Neoplasia

Leishmaniasis in endemic areas

Hyperthyroidism (cats)

Dermatomyositis

Drug or vaccine reaction

Pulmonary bronchiolar adenocarcinoma (lung-digit syndrome, cats)

## FUNGAL CLAW INFECTION

Typically caused by dermatophytes

*Microsporum canis* (cats)

*Trichophyton mentagrophytes* (dogs)

*Microsporum gypseum* and *Candida* less common

*Malassezia* (dogs and cats)

## SYMMETRICAL LUPOID ONYCHODYSTROPHY

Suspected to be immune-mediated. German Shepherds and Rottweilers may be predisposed. Acute onset of claw loss, initially 1–2, but eventually, all claws slough. Replacement claws are misshapen, soft or brittle, discolored, and friable, and usually slough again. Feet are painful and pruritic. Paronychia is uncommon unless secondary bacterial infection is present.

## DRUG ERUPTION

## VASCULITIS

## Diagnostic Tests for Abnormal Claws

Cytology—suppurative to pyogranulomatous inflammation with bacteria.

Bacterial culture of exudates from claw or claw fold.

Mixed infections common. *Staphylococcus* spp. usually isolated.

Fungal culture—*Trichophyton* spp. most commonly isolated, but may also see *Microsporum* spp. or *Malassezia* spp.

Radiography—rule out osteomyelitis.

Dermatohistopathology—(P3 amputation) only recommended to rule out neoplasia. With symmetric lupoid onychodystrophy, see basal cell hydropic degeneration, degeneration or apoptosis of individual keratinocytes in the basal layer, pigmentary incontinence, and lichenoid interface dermatitis. Systemic lupoid onychodystrophy is most commonly diagnosed by typical history and clinical signs along with ruling out other differentials.

## Erosions and Ulcerations of Skin or Mucous Membranes

## Differential Diagnosis, Dogs

### EXCORIATION FROM ANY PRURITIC SKIN DISEASE

### INFECTION

*Bacterial Pyoderma*

Surface (pyotraumatic moist dermatitis, intertrigo)

Deep (folliculitis, furunculosis, bacterial stomatitis)

*Fungal*

Yeast infection (*Malassezia pachydermatis, Candida* spp.)

Dermatophytosis

Systemic fungal infection (blastomycosis, coccidioidomycosis, cryptococcosis, histoplasmosis, others)

Subcutaneous mycoses (pythiosis, zygomycosis, phaeohyphomycosis, sporotrichosis, eumycotic mycetoma, others)

*Parasitic*

Demodicosis

*Neoplasia*

Squamous cell carcinoma

Epitheliotropic lymphoma

*Metabolic Derangements*

Uremia/renal failure

Necrolytic migratory erythema

Calcinosis cutis (hyperadrenocorticism)

*Physical/Chemical Injury*

Drug reactions

Urine scald

Thermal injury (burn, freeze)

Solar injury

*Immune-Mediated Disorders*

Discoid lupus erythematosus (DLE)

Pemphigus

Uveodermatologic syndrome

Miscellaneous autoimmune subepidermal vesiculobullous diseases (bullous pemphigoid, epidermolysis acquisita, linear IgA bullous disease, mucocutaneous pemphigoid, bullous systemic lupus-type 1)

*Miscellaneous*

Arthropod bites

Dermatomyositis

Dystrophic epidermolysis bullosa, junctional epidermolysis bullosa

Idiopathic ulceration of Collies

Toxic epidermal necrolysis, erythema multiforme (EM)

## Differential Diagnosis, Cats

### INFECTION

*Viral*

Calicivirus

Herpesvirus

*Bacterial*

Atypical mycobacteriosis

*Fungal*

Cryptococcosis

Systemic and subcutaneous mycoses

Sporotrichosis

### NEOPLASIA

Squamous cell carcinomas (especially white outdoor cats)

Fibrosarcoma

Cutaneous lymphoma

### METABOLIC DERANGEMENTS

Uremia/renal disease

### PHYSICAL/CHEMICAL INJURY

Thermal

Drug reactions

### IMMUNE-MEDIATED DISORDERS

Bullous pemphigoid

Pemphigus foliaceus

Plasma cell pododermatitis

Toxic epidermal necrolysis

### INFLAMMATORY/ALLERGIC DISORDERS

Eosinophilic plaque

Indolent ulcer

Arthropod bites

### MISCELLANEOUS/IDIOPATHIC

Dystrophic epidermolysis bullosa

Idiopathic ulceration of dorsal neck

Junctional epidermolysis bullosa

## Folliculitis

## Differential Diagnosis

## Superficial Folliculitis

Inflammation of hair follicles

- Bacterial pyoderma

- Fungal (dermatophytosis)
- Parasitic (demodicosis, *Pelodera* dermatitis)

## Deep Folliculitis/Furunculosis

Inflammation of hair follicles with subsequent follicular rupture into dermis and subcutaneous tissues
- Deep pyodermas

## Otitis Externa, Chronic

## Primary Causes

### ALLERGY
Atopy
Adverse reactions to foods
Contact dermatitis

### PARASITES
*Otodectes cynotis*
*Notoedres cati*
*Sarcoptes scabiei*
*Demodex* spp.
Chiggers
Flies
Ticks (spinous ear tick)

### DERMATOPHYTES

### ENDOCRINE DISORDERS

### HYPOTHYROIDISM

### FOREIGN BODIES
Foxtails, hair, etc.

### GLANDULAR CONDITIONS
Ceruminous gland hyperplasia
Sebaceous gland hyperplasia or hypoplasia
Altered type or rate of secretions

### AUTOIMMUNE DISEASES
Systemic lupus erythematosus (SLE)
Pemphigus foliaceus/erythematosus
Cold agglutinin disease
Juvenile cellulitis

### VIRUSES
Distemper

### MISCELLANEOUS
Solar dermatitis
Frostbite

Vasculitis/vasculopathy
Eosinophilic dermatitis
Sterile eosinophilic folliculitis
Relapsing polychondritis

## Predisposing Factors

### CONFORMATION
Stenotic canals
Hair in canals
Pendulous pinnae
Hairy, concave pinna

### EXCESSIVE MOISTURE
Swimmer's ear
High-humidity climate

### EXCESSIVE CERUMEN PRODUCTION
Secondary to underlying disease
Primary (idiopathic)

### TREATMENT EFFECTS
Trauma from cotton swabs
Topical irritants
Superinfections from altering microflora

### OBSTRUCTIVE EAR DISEASE
Polyps
Granulomas
Tumors

### SYSTEMIC DISEASE
Immunosuppression
Debilitation
Negative catabolic states

## Perpetuating Factors

### BACTERIA (MOST COMMONLY *STAPHYLOCOCCUS SPP.*, *STREPTOCOCCUS SPP.*, *PSEUDOMONAS SPP.*, *PROTEUS*, *ESCHERICHIA COLI*)

### YEAST (*MALASSEZIA PACHYDERMATIS*)

### PROGRESSIVE PATHOLOGIC CHANGES
Hyperkeratosis
Hyperplasia
Epithelial folds
Apocrine gland hypertrophy
Hidradenitis
Fibrosis

### OTITIS MEDIA
Purulent
Caseated or keratinous
Cholesteatoma
Proliferative
Destructive osteomyelitis

## Parasitic Dermatoses

## Classification

### FLEAS (*CTENOCEPHALIDES FELIS* MOST COMMON)
Flea infestation
Flea allergy dermatitis
- Caudal distribution of lesions (dogs)
- Miliary dermatitis (cats)

### DEMODICOSIS
Dog (*Demodex canis, Demodex injai, Demodex cornei*)
Cat (*Demodex cati, Demodex gatoi*)

### SARCOPTIC MANGE
*Sarcoptes scabiei* (dogs, rarely cats)
*Notoedres cati* (cats, rarely dogs)

### EAR MITES
*Otodectes cynotis* (common in both dogs and cats)

### CHEYLETIELLOSIS
*Cheyletiella yasguri* (primary host is dogs)
*C. blakei* (primary host is cats)
*C. parasitovorax* (primary host is rabbits)
All *Cheyletiella* species freely contagious from one
species to another

### CHIGGERS
Larval stage (six-legged, bright red or orange) is the
parasitic stage; nymph and adult are free living.

### TICKS
Brown dog tick (*Rhipicephalus sanguineus*)
American dog tick (*Dermacentor variabilis*)
Rocky Mountain wood tick (*Dermacentor andersoni*)
Lone star tick (*Amblyomma americanum*)
Deer tick *(Ixodes dammini):* primary vector of *Borrelia
burgdorferi*
Spinous ear tick *(Otobius megnini)*

### LICE
Sucking lice of dogs (*Linognathus setosus*)
Biting lice of dogs (*Trichodectes canis, Heterodoxus spinger*)
Lice of cats (*Felicola subrostrata*)

### INSECTS OF ORDER DIPTERA

Mosquitoes: eosinophilic dermatitis (especially cats)

Black flies, stable flies, horn flies, houseflies: attack ear pinnae of dogs

Myiasis (development of fly larvae in skin or hair coat): screwworm, blow flies, flesh flies

*Cuterebra* fly larva

### HELMINTH PARASITES

Hookworm dermatitis *(Ancylostoma, Uncinaria)*

Pelodera dermatitis *(Pelodera strongyloides)*

Dracunculiasis *(Dracunculus insignis)*

## Pigmentation

## Differential Diagnosis for Changes in Skin Pigmentation

### HYPOPIGMENTATION

Vitiligo (Belgian Tervuren, Rottweiler, Doberman Pinscher, Newfoundland, Collie, German Shorthaired Pointer, Old English Sheepdog, Siamese cat)

Uveodermatologic syndrome (northern breeds such as Siberian Husky, Samoyed, Akita)

Acquired idiopathic hypopigmentation of nose (Labrador Retriever, Golden Retriever, Malamute, Siberian Husky, Samoyed, Poodle, German Shepherd)

DLE (German Shepherd, Collie, others)

Dermatomyositis (Collie, Shetland Sheepdog, Beauceron Shepherd)

### HYPERPIGMENTATION

*Postinflammatory Hyperpigmentation*

Any Chronic Pruritic Skin Disease

Atopy

Adverse food reactions

Pyoderma

*Malassezia* dermatitis

Sarcoptic mange

EM

Many others

*Demodicosis*

*Endocrinopathies*

Hypothyroidism

Hyperadrenocorticism

Hyperestrogenism

*Dermatophytosis*

*Nevus*

*Lentigo*

*Lentigo simplex in orange cats*

*Acanthosis nigricans (Dachshunds)*

*Alopecia X*
Recurrent flank alopecia
Sun exposure/burns

*Feline acromelanism*

*Urticaria pigmentosa (Sphinx cats)*

*Neoplasia (Melanoma)*

## Pyoderma

## Differential Diagnosis

### SURFACE PYODERMA
Pyotraumatic dermatitis (acute moist dermatitis, "hot spot")
Intertrigo (skin fold dermatitis)

### SUPERFICIAL PYODERMA
Impetigo (subcorneal pustules of sparsely haired skin)
- Puppy pyoderma
Bullous impetigo
- Hyperadrenocorticism, hypothyroidism, diabetes mellitus
Mucocutaneous pyoderma
- Dogs (German Shepherds predisposed)
Superficial bacterial folliculitis
- *Staphylococcus pseudintermedius* most common
- Local trauma secondary to pruritus (allergy, fleas, scabies, demodicosis, etc.)
Dermatophilosis (rare, actinomycotic superficial crusting dermatitis)
Methicillin-resistant *Staphylococcus pseudintermedius*

### DEEP PYODERMA
Always secondary to predisposing problem
Localized lesion (laceration, penetrating wound, animal bite, foreign body)
Generalized (suspect underlying systemic disease)
Clinical syndromes associated with deep pyoderma
- Deep folliculitis, furunculosis, cellulitis
- Pyotraumatic folliculitis, furunculosis

- Nasal folliculitis, furunculosis
- Muzzle folliculitis and furunculosis
- Pododermatitis (interdigital pyoderma)
- German Shepherd Dog folliculitis, furunculosis, cellulitis
- Acral lick furunculosis
- Aerobic cellulitis
- Anaerobic cellulitis
- Subcutaneous abscesses
- Bacterial pseudomycetoma
- Mycobacterial granulomas
  - Cutaneous tuberculosis (*Mycobacterium tuberculosis, M. bovis*)
  - Feline leprosy (*M. lepraemurium*)
  - Opportunistic mycobacterial granulomas
- Actinomycosis
- Actinobacillosis
- Nocardiosis
- Cats: bite wounds, cellulitis, abscess, feline acne

## MISCELLANEOUS BACTERIAL INFECTIONS

Brucellosis, plague, borreliosis, *Trichomycosis axillaris*, L-form infections

# Endocrinologic and Metabolic Disorders

## Acromegaly

In dogs, acromegaly is caused by endogenous progesterone from the luteal phase of the estrous cycle or by exogenous progesterone used for estrous prevention. Elevated progesterone, in turn, stimulates excessive growth hormone secretion of mammary origin. In cats, acromegaly is caused by a pituitary adenoma, usually a macroadenoma, which secretes excessive amounts of growth hormone. Physical changes are less pronounced in cats than in dogs.

### Clinical Findings, Dogs

Hypertrophy of mouth, tongue, and pharynx
Thick skin folds, myxedema, hypertrichosis
Prognathism
Wide interdental spacing
Visceral organomegaly
Insulin-resistant diabetes mellitus
Polyuria

Polyphagia

Elevated alkaline phosphatase (ALP)

## Clinical Findings, Cats

Physical changes most pronounced on head, but all the physical changes listed for dogs may be seen.

Insulin-resistant diabetes mellitus (severe)

Degenerative arthropathy/lameness

Polyuria/polydipsia

Polyphagia

Panting

Lethargy/exercise intolerance

Dyspnea secondary to hypertrophic cardiomyopathy and heart failure

Neurologic signs when macroadenoma becomes large

- Lethargy, stupor
- Adipsia
- Anorexia
- Temperature deregulation
- Circling
- Seizures
- Pituitary dysfunction
  - Hypogonadism
  - Hypothyroidism
  - Hypoadrenocorticism (feline acromegaly may also coexist with pituitary-dependent hyperadrenocorticism)

## Adrenal Tumors

### Differential Diagnosis

#### NONFUNCTIONAL ADRENAL TUMOR (DOG, RARELY CAT)

No hormone secreted

Diagnosis by exclusion

Histopathology

#### FUNCTIONAL ADRENOCORTICAL TUMOR

*Cortisol-Secreting Tumor*

Hyperadrenocorticism (Cushing syndrome) (dog, rarely cat)

Diagnosis by adrenocorticotropic hormone (ACTH) stimulation test, low-dose dexamethasone suppression test, adrenal ultrasound, CT scan

*Aldosterone-Secreting Tumor*

Hyperaldosteronism (Conn syndrome) (cat, rarely dog)

Diagnosis by assessing Na/K, ACTH stimulation test (measure aldosterone)

*Progesterone-Secreting Tumor*
Mimics hyperadrenocorticism (cat, less commonly dog)
Diagnosis by measuring serum progesterone

*Steroid Hormone Precursor–Secreting Tumor*
17-hydroxyprogesterone
Mimics hyperadrenocorticism (dog)
Diagnosis by ACTH stimulation test (measure steroid hormone precursors)
Deoxycorticosterone
Mimics hyperadrenocorticism (dog)
Diagnosis by ACTH stimulation test (measure steroid hormone precursors)

## FUNCTIONAL ADRENOMEDULLARY TUMOR
*Epinephrine-Secreting Tumor*
Pheochromocytosis (dog, rarely cat)
Diagnosis by exclusion, histopathology

## Congenital Hypothyroidism (Hypothyroidism in Puppies)
### Clinical Findings

Dwarfism
Short, broad skull with short, thick neck
Enlarged cranium
Shortened limbs
Shortened mandible
Mental dullness
Alopecia
Retention of puppy coat
Kyphosis
Inappetence
Hypothermia
Constipation
Gait abnormalities
Delayed dental eruption
Macroglossia
Dry coat
Thick skin
Lethargy
Dyspnea
Goiter

## Diabetes Insipidus

## Differential Diagnosis

Features of diabetes insipidus include polyuria, polydipsia, and a near-continuous demand for water. Only the following three disorders can cause the degree of polyuria and dilute urine seen with diabetes insipidus:

- Central diabetes insipidus
- Nephrogenic diabetes insipidus
- Primary polydipsia

## Causes in Dogs and Cats

### CENTRAL DIABETES INSIPIDUS

Idiopathic

Traumatic

Neoplasia

- Primary pituitary neoplasm
- Meningioma
- Craniopharyngioma
- Chromophobe adenoma
- Chromophobe adenocarcinoma
- Metastatic neoplasia

Pituitary and hypothalamic malformation

Cysts

Inflammation

Parasitic lesions

Complication of pituitary surgery (hypophysectomy)

Familial?

### NEPHROGENIC DIABETES INSIPIDUS

*Polyuria caused by nonresponsiveness to antidiuretic hormone (ADH)*

Primary idiopathic

Primary familial (Siberian Husky)

Secondary acquired

- Renal insufficiency or failure
- Hyperadrenocorticism
- Hypoadrenocorticism
- Hepatic insufficiency
- Pyometra
- Hypercalcemia
- Hypokalemia
- Postobstructive diuresis
- Diabetes mellitus
- Normoglycemic glucosuria

- Hyperthyroidism
- Iatrogenic or drug-induced
- Renal medullary solute washout

## Diabetic Ketoacidosis

### Clinical Findings

No signs may be seen early with diabetic ketoacidosis.

#### HISTORICAL FINDINGS
Lethargy
Anorexia
Vomiting

#### PHYSICAL EXAMINATION FINDINGS
Dehydration
Depression
Weakness
Tachypnea
Vomiting
Acetone odor on breath
Slow, deep breaths (secondary to metabolic acidosis)
Abdominal pain/abdominal distension secondary to concurrent pancreatitis

#### CLINICOPATHOLOGIC FINDINGS
Hyperglycemia
Neutrophilic leukocytosis
Hemoconcentration
Metabolic acidosis (decreased total carbon dioxide concentration)
Hypercholesterolemia/lipemia
Increased ALP
Increased ALT
Increased blood urea nitrogen (BUN)/creatinine
Hyponatremia
Hypochloremia
Hypokalemia
Hypophosphatemia
Hypomagnesemia
Increased amylase/lipase
Hyperosmolality
Glycosuria
Ketonuria
Urinary tract infection

## Diabetes Mellitus

### Potential Factors in Etiopathogenesis

Obesity
Pancreatitis
Immune-mediated insulitis
Concurrent hormonal disease
- Hyperadrenocorticism
- Diestrus-induced excess of growth hormone
- Hypothyroidism
Genetics (dog, possibly cat)
Drugs
- Glucocorticoids
- Megestrol acetate (cat)
- Thiazide diuretics
- Beta-adrenergic agonists
Infection
Concurrent illness
- Renal insufficiency
- Cardiac disease
Hyperlipidemia (dog, possibly cat)
Islet amyloidosis

### Clinicopathologic Abnormalities, Uncomplicated Diabetes Mellitus

#### CBC

Often normal
Leukocytosis if pancreatitis or infection present

#### SERUM CHEMISTRY

Hyperglycemia
Mild increase in ALP and ALT
Hypercholesterolemia/hypertriglyceridemia

#### URINALYSIS

Urine specific gravity normal to mildly decreased
(>1.025)
Glycosuria
Variable ketonuria
Bacteriuria
Proteinuria

#### ANCILLARY TESTS

Increased amylase/lipase if pancreatitis present
Normal serum trypsin-like immunoreactivity (TLI)
Low TLI with exocrine pancreatic insufficiency
High TLI with acute pancreatitis
Normal-to-high TLI with chronic pancreatitis

Low-to-normal serum insulin with insulin-dependent diabetes mellitus

Low, normal, or increased serum insulin with non–insulin-dependent diabetes mellitus

## Potential Complications

### COMMON

Iatrogenic hypoglycemia
Polyuria/polydipsia
Weight loss
Cataracts (dog)
Anterior uveitis
Bacterial infections (especially urinary tract infection [UTI])
Ketoacidosis
Pancreatitis
Peripheral neuropathy (cat)
Hepatic lipidosis

### UNCOMMON

Peripheral neuropathy (dog)
Glomerulopathy
Glomerulosclerosis
Retinopathy
Exocrine pancreatic insufficiency (EPI)
Gastric paresis
Diabetic diarrhea
Diabetic dermatopathy

## Causes of Insulin Resistance or Ineffectiveness in Dogs and Cats

### CAUSED BY INSULIN THERAPY

Improper administration
Inadequate dose
Inactive insulin
Diluted insulin
Somogyi effect
Inappropriate insulin administration
Impaired insulin absorption
Antiinsulin antibody excess

### CAUSED BY CONCURRENT DISORDER

Obesity
Diabetogenic drugs
Hyperadrenocorticism
Hypothyroidism (dog)
Hyperthyroidism (cat)

UTI
Oral infections
Chronic inflammation/pancreatitis
Diestrus (bitch)
Acromegaly (cat)
Renal insufficiency
Hepatic insufficiency
Cardiac insufficiency
Glucagonoma
Pheochromocytoma
EPI
Hyperlipidemia
Neoplasia

## Clinical Findings Associated With Insulin-Secreting Tumors

Seizures
Weakness
Collapse
Ataxia
Polyphagia
Weight gain
Muscle fasciculations
Posterior weakness (neuropathy)
Lethargy
Nervousness
Unusual behavior

## Gastrinoma (Zollinger-Ellison Syndrome)

### Clinical Findings

#### CLINICAL SIGNS
Vomiting
Weight loss
Anorexia
Diarrhea
Gastric and duodenal ulceration
Hematochezia
Hematemesis
Melena
Obstipation
Lethargy/depression
Abdominal pain
Esophageal pain and ulceration
Regurgitation

Fever
Polydipsia
Thin body condition
Pallor

### CLINICOPATHOLOGIC FINDINGS

Regenerative anemia
Hypoproteinemia
Neutrophilic leukocytosis
Hypoalbuminemia
Hypocalcemia
Mild increases in hepatic enzymes
Hypochloremia
Hypokalemia
Hyponatremia
Metabolic acidosis
Metabolic acidosis (secondary to vomiting)
Hyperglycemia, hypoglycemia (uncommon)

## Glucagonoma

## Clinical Findings in Dogs

### CLINICAL SIGNS

Necrolytic migratory erythema (crusting skin rash of
elbows, hocks, nose, scrotum, flank, ventral abdomen,
distal extremities, and mucocutaneous junctions of
mouth, eyes, prepuce, and vulva)
Footpad lesions
Glucose intolerance/diabetes mellitus (caused by excess
glycogenolysis and gluconeogenesis)
Oral ulcerations
Lethargy
Weight loss
Decreased appetite
Muscle atrophy
Peripheral lymphadenopathy

### CLINICOPATHOLOGIC FINDINGS

Hyperglycemia
Nonregenerative anemia
Increased hepatic enzymes
Decreased albumin
Decreased globulin
Decreased BUN
Decreased cholesterol
Glucosuria
Abdominal ultrasound lesions

- Increased echogenicity of portal and hepatic vein walls
- Diffuse hyperechogenicity
- Multiple small hypoechoic foci

## Hyperadrenocorticism

### Clinical Findings

#### POTENTIAL CLINICAL SIGNS

Polyuria/polydipsia
Alopecia
Pendulous abdomen
Hepatomegaly
Polyphagia
Muscle weakness
Muscle atrophy
Pyoderma
Comedones
Panting
Pacing/restlessness
Hyperpigmentation
Systemic hypertension
Testicular atrophy
Anestrus
Calcinosis cutis
Facial nerve paralysis
Pulmonary thromboembolism
Ligament/tendon injury

#### POTENTIAL CLINICOPATHOLOGIC FINDINGS

UTI/pyelonephritis
Decreased urine specific gravity
Increased serum ALP
Increased ALT
Hypercholesterolemia
Hypertriglyceridemia
Hyperglycemia (mild to moderate)
Diabetes mellitus (uncommon)
Increased serum bile acids
Decreased BUN and creatinine (secondary to diuresis)
Hypophosphatemia
Stress leukogram
- Neutrophilia
- Lymphopenia
- Eosinopenia
- Monocytosis

Thrombocytosis
Mild erythrocytosis
Decreased total serum thyroxine ($T_4$) or free $T_4$
Urolithiasis

## Hyperglycemia

### Differential Diagnosis

Diabetes mellitus
Stress (physiologic in cat)
Hyperadrenocorticism
Drug therapy
- Glucocorticoids
- Progestogens
- Megestrol acetate
- Thiazide diuretics

Dextrose-containing fluids
Parenteral nutrition
Postprandial effect (diets containing monosaccharides, disaccharides, propylene glycol)
Exocrine pancreatic neoplasia
Pancreatitis
Renal insufficiency
Acromegaly (cat)
Pheochromocytoma (dog)
Diestrus (bitch)
Head trauma

## Hypoadrenocorticism

### Potential Clinical Findings

#### CLINICAL SIGNS

Lethargy/depression
Episodic weakness
Vomiting
Anorexia
Waxing and waning illness
Weight loss/failure to gain weight
Bradycardia
Dehydration/hypovolemia
Diarrhea
Polyuria or polydipsia
Collapse
Syncope
Restlessness/shaking/shivering

Regurgitation

Muscle cramping

GI hemorrhage/melena

Abdominal pain

## POTENTIAL CLINICOPATHOLOGIC FINDINGS

Hyponatremia

Hyperkalemia

Hypochloremia

Decreased sodium/potassium ratio (<24:1)

Azotemia (prerenal)

- Increased BUN
- Increased creatinine
- Increased phosphate

Decreased bicarbonate and total $CO_2$ concentrations

Hypercalcemia

Hypoglycemia

Hypoalbuminemia

Increased hepatic enzymes

Metabolic acidosis

Lymphocytosis

Eosinophilia

Relative neutropenia

Anemia (usually nonregenerative)

Variable urine specific gravity (<1.030)

## Hypoglycemia

### Differential Diagnosis

#### EXCESS SECRETION OF INSULIN OR INSULIN-LIKE FACTORS

Insulinoma (beta-cell tumor)

Extrapancreatic tumor (hepatocellular carcinoma, hepatoma, leiomyosarcoma, leiomyoma)

Islet cell hyperplasia

#### DECREASED GLUCOSE PRODUCTION

Toy breeds

Neonates

Hunting dog hypoglycemia

Malnutrition

Pregnancy

Fasting/starvation

Hypoadrenocorticism

Hypopituitarism

Growth hormone deficiency

Liver disease (portosystemic shunt, chronic fibrosis/cirrhosis)

Glycogen storage diseases

## EXCESS GLUCOSE CONSUMPTION
Sepsis
Extreme exercise
Severe erythrocytosis

## DRUG-ASSOCIATED CAUSES
Insulin
Oral hypoglycemics
Ethanol, ethylene glycol
Many other drugs reported to cause hypoglycemia
in humans

## SPURIOUS
Blood cells not promptly separated from serum
Glucometers, laboratory error

## Hyponatremia/hyperkalemia

## Differential Diagnosis

### HYPOADRENOCORTICISM

### RENAL OR URINARY TRACT DISEASE
Urethral obstruction
Acute renal failure
Chronic oliguric or anuric renal failure
Postobstructive diuresis
Nephrotic syndrome

### SEVERE GASTROINTESTINAL DISEASE
Parasitic infestation
- Whipworm (trichuriasis)
- Roundworm (ascariasis)
- Hookworm (ancylostomiasis)
Salmonellosis
Viral enteritis
- Parvovirus
- Canine distemper virus
Gastric dilatation/volvulus
GI perforation
Severe malabsorption
Hemorrhagic gastroenteritis
Pancreatic disease

### SEVERE HEPATIC FAILURE
Cirrhosis
Neoplasia

## SEVERE METABOLIC OR RESPIRATORY ACIDOSIS

## CONGESTIVE HEART FAILURE

## MASSIVE RELEASE OF POTASSIUM INTO EXTRACELLULAR FLUID

Crush injury
Aortic thrombosis
Rhabdomyolysis
- heat stroke
- Exertional

Massive sepsis
Massive hemolysis

## PLEURAL EFFUSION

## PREGNANCY

## LYMPHANGIOSARCOMA

## PSEUDOHYPERKALEMIA

Akitas and related breeds
Severe leukocytosis (>100,000/mm$^3$)
Severe thrombocytosis (>1 million/mm$^3$)

## DIABETES MELLITUS

## PRIMARY POLYDIPSIA

## INAPPROPRIATE ADH SECRETION

## DRUG-INDUCED

Potassium-sparing diuretics
Nonsteroidal antiinflammatory drugs (NSAIDs)
Angiotensin-converting enzyme (ACE) inhibitors
Potassium-containing fluids

## Insulinoma

### Differential Diagnosis for Insulin-Secreting B-Cell Neoplasia

#### EXCESS INSULIN OR INSULIN-LIKE FACTORS

Insulinoma
Extrapancreatic tumor
Islet cell hyperplasia

#### DECREASED GLUCOSE PRODUCTION

Hypoadrenocorticism
Hypopituitarism
Growth hormone deficiency
Liver disease

Glycogen storage diseases
Neonates
Toy breeds
Fasting
Malnutrition
Pregnancy
Uremia

### EXCESS GLUCOSE CONSUMPTION
Sepsis
Extreme exercise

### DRUG-ASSOCIATED CAUSES
Insulin
Oral hypoglycemics (sulfonylurea)
Salicylates (e.g., aspirin)
Acetaminophen
β-blockers
β$_2$-agonists
Ethanol
Xylitol
Monoamine oxidase inhibitors
Tricyclic antidepressants
ACE inhibitors
Antibiotics (e.g., tetracycline)
Lidocaine overdose
Lithium

### FACTITIOUS HYPOGLYCEMIA
Failure to separate blood cells from serum promptly
Severe polycythemia or leukocytosis when serum
separation delayed

## Parathyroidism

## Hyperparathyroidism, Primary—Clinical Findings

### CLINICAL SIGNS
Polyuria/polydipsia
Weight loss
Anorexia
Lethargy, listlessness
UTI
Urolithiasis (pollakiuria, stranguria, hematuria)
Vomiting
Constipation
Mental dullness, obtundation, coma
Weakness, muscle wasting, shivering

## CLINICOPATHOLOGIC FINDINGS
Hypercalcemia
Increased ionized calcemia
Low normal to low serum phosphorus
Decreased urine specific gravity
Hematuria
Pyuria
Crystalluria
Bacteriuria

## Hypoparathyroidism—Clinical Findings

### CLINICAL SIGNS
Seizures
Splinted abdomen
Stiff gait
Intermittent lameness
Muscle fasciculations, cramping, tremors
Facial rubbing, biting at feet
Fever
Paroxysmal tachyarrhythmias
Muffled heart sounds
Weak pulses
Disorientation
Behavioral changes (restless, nervous, anxious,
   aggressive)

### CLINICOPATHOLOGIC FINDINGS
Hypocalcemia
Hyperphosphatemia
Decreased serum parathyroid hormone (PTH)
   concentration
Low normal-to-low PTH with low ionized calcium
   consistent with hypoparathyroidism diagnosis

### ELECTROCARDIOGRAPHIC FINDINGS
Deep, wide T waves
Prolonged QT interval
Bradycardia

## Pheochromocytoma

## Clinical Findings
Intermittent weakness
Intermittent collapse
Panting
Tachypnea
Seizures

Acute blindness
Tachycardia
Lethargy
Inappetence
Cardiac arrhythmias
Restlessness
Exercise intolerance
Panting/tachypnea
Weak pulses
Vomiting
Diarrhea
Weight loss
Muscle wasting
Polyuria/polydipsia
Abdominal distension
Rear limb edema
Pale mucous membranes
Abdominal pain
Hemorrhage (epistaxis, surgical incision sites)
Palpable abdominal mass
Sudden death

## Pituitary Dwarfism

### Clinical Findings

#### MUSCULOSKELETAL SIGNS
Stunted growth
Delayed growth plate closure
Thin skeleton
Immature facial features
Square, chunky contour as adult
Bone deformities
Delayed dental eruption

#### DERMATOLOGIC SIGNS
Soft, woolly hair coat
Lack of guard hairs
Alopecia (bilaterally symmetric trunk, neck, and
  proximal extremities)
Hyperpigmentation
Thin, fragile skin
Wrinkles
Scales
Comedones
Papules
Pyoderma

Seborrhea sicca
Retention of secondary hairs

### REPRODUCTIVE SIGNS
Testicular atrophy
Unilateral or bilateral cryptorchidism
Flaccid penile sheath
Failure to have estrous cycles

### OTHER SIGNS
Mental dullness
Shrill, puppylike bark
Signs of secondary hypothyroidism
Signs of secondary adrenal insufficiency

## Thyroid Disease

## Hyperthyroidism, Feline—Clinical Findings

### CLINICAL SIGNS
Weight loss/thin body condition
Polyphagia
Hyperactivity
Palpable thyroid nodule (goiter)
Tachycardia
Vomiting
Cardiac murmur
Premature beats
Gallop rhythm
Aggressiveness
Panting
Pacing
Restlessness
Increased nail growth
Alopecia
Polyuria/polydipsia
Diarrhea
Increased fecal volume
Muscle weakness
CHF
Dyspnea
Retinal lesions (tortuous blood vessels retinal tears, retinal detachment)
Ventroflexion of neck
Unkempt coat/alopecia
Tremor
Weakness
Anorexia
Heat avoidance

## Hypothyroidism, Canine—Clinical Findings

### CLINICAL SIGNS

Lethargy/exercise intolerance

Weight gain

Cold intolerance

Mental dullness

Dermatologic signs

- Alopecia
- Superficial pyoderma
- Seborrhea sicca or oleosa
- Dry, scaly skin
- Changes in hair coat quality and color
- Hyperkeratosis
- Hyperpigmentation
- Comedones
- Hypertrichosis
- Ceruminous otitis
- Myxedema (cutaneous mucinosis)
- Poor wound healing
- Slow regrowth of hair

Reproductive abnormalities

- Male: decreased libido, testicular atrophy, hypospermia
- Female: delayed estrus, silent estrus, failure to cycle, abortion, small litters, uterine inertia, weak or still-born puppies

Peripheral neuropathies

- Generalized peripheral neuropathies
- Specific peripheral neuropathies (especially cranial nerves [CNs], facial, trigeminal, vestibulocochlear)

Cerebral dysfunction (myxedema coma [rare])

Cardiovascular signs

- Sinus bradycardia, weak apex beat, low QRS voltages, inverted T waves, hypercholesterolemia leading to atherosclerosis (rare)

Ocular abnormalities (corneal lipidosis, corneal ulceration, uveitis, secondary glaucoma, lipemia retinalis, retinal detachment, and keratoconjunctivitis sicca reported, but causal relationship not proven)

Congenital hypothyroidism-severe signs (see Congenital Hypothyroidism)

### CLINICOPATHOLOGIC CHANGES

Nonregenerative anemia

Hypercholesterolemia

Hypertriglyceridemia

Mild increases in hepatic enzymes

# Gastroenterologic Disorders

## Chronic Constipation, Feline

### Differential Diagnosis

#### NEUROMUSCULAR DYSFUNCTION
Colonic smooth muscle: idiopathic megacolon, aging
Spinal cord disease: lumbosacral disease, cauda equina syndrome, sacral spinal cord deformities (Manx cat)
Hypogastric or pelvic nerve disorders: traumatic injury, malignancy, dysautonomia

#### MECHANICAL OBSTRUCTION
Intraluminal: foreign material, neoplasia, rectal diverticula, perineal hernia, anorectal strictures
Intramural: neoplasia
Extraluminal: pelvic fractures, neoplasia

#### INFLAMMATION
Perianal fistula, proctitis, anal sac abscess, anorectal foreign bodies, perianal bite wounds

#### METABOLIC AND ENDOCRINE
Metabolic: dehydration, hypokalemia, hypercalcemia
Endocrine: hypothyroidism, obesity, nutritional secondary hyperparathyroidism

### ENVIRONMENTAL AND BEHAVIORAL

Soiled litter box, inactivity, hospitalization, change in environment

### DRUG ADMINISTRATION

Opioids, anticholinergics

## Dental and Oral Cavity Diseases

### Differential Diagnosis

#### TRAUMA

Fractures
- Crown
- Root
- Mandible
- Maxilla

Avulsion

Pulp injury

Temporomandibular luxation

#### CARIES

#### FELINE DENTAL RESORPTIVE LESIONS

#### PERIODONTAL DISEASE

Gingivitis

Gingival recession

Bone loss, osteomyelitis

Tooth loss

Gingival hyperplasia

#### TOOTH ROOT ABSCESS

#### ORONASAL FISTULA

#### STOMATITIS (FAUCITIS, GLOSSITIS, PHARYNGITIS)

FIV, FeLV, feline syncytium-forming virus

Immune-mediated disease related to plaque bacteria

Feline calicivirus, feline herpesvirus, FIP

Candidiasis

Uremia

Trauma (foreign objects, caustic agents, electric cord bite)

Autoimmune disease (pemphigus, lupus, idiopathic vasculitis, toxic epidermal necrolysis)

Feline idiopathic gingivitis/pharyngitis

#### NEOPLASIA

*Malignant*

Fibrosarcoma

Squamous cell carcinoma

Melanoma
Salivary gland neoplasms

*Benign*
Epulis
- Fibromatous
- Acanthomatous
- Ossifying

Papilloma
Fibroma
Lipoma
Chondroma
Osteoma
Hemangioma
Hemangiopericytoma
Histiocytoma

## EOSINOPHILIC GRANULOMA COMPLEX

Linear granuloma
Eosinophilic ulcer (usually on maxillary lips)

## SIALOCELE

# Diarrhea

## Causes of Diarrhea

### GASTROINTESTINAL DISEASE

Diffuse GI disease (e.g., inflammation or lymphoma)
Gastric disease (achlorhydria, dumping syndromes)
Intestinal disease (primary small intestinal disease, primary large intestinal disease, dietary induced such as food poisoning, gluttony, or sudden change of diet)

### NONGASTROINTESTINAL DISEASE

Pancreatic disease (EPI, pancreatitis, pancreatic carcinoma, gastrinoma, or Zollinger-Ellison syndrome)
Liver disease (hepatocellular failure, intrahepatic and extrahepatic cholestasis)
Endocrine disease (classical hypoadrenocorticism, atypical hypoadrenocorticism, hyperthyroidism, hypothyroidism)
Renal disease (uremia, nephrotic syndrome)
Polysystemic infection (e.g., distemper, leptospirosis, infectious canine hepatitis in dogs, FIP, FeLV, FIV in cats)
Miscellaneous (toxemias such as pyometra and peritonitis, CHF, autoimmune disease, metastatic neoplasia, various toxins and drugs)

## Classification of Diarrhea

### MECHANISTIC
Secretory
Osmotic
Permeability (exudative)
Dysmotility
Mixed

### TEMPORAL
Acute
Chronic

### ANATOMIC
Extraintestinal
Small intestinal
Large intestinal
Diffuse

### PATHOPHYSIOLOGIC
Biochemical
Allergic
Inflammatory
Neoplastic

### ETIOLOGIC
Bacteria
Dietary
Fungal
Idiopathic
Parasitic
Viral

### CAUSAL
EPI, salmonellosis, lymphoma, other

### CLINICAL
Acute, nonfatal, mild, self-limiting
Acute, severe potentially fatal
Acute systemic disease
Chronic
Chronic protein-losing

## Differentiation of Small Intestinal Diarrhea from Large Intestinal Diarrhea

### SMALL INTESTINAL DIARRHEA SIGNS
Weight loss with chronicity
Polyphagia sometimes
Normal to slightly increased frequency of bowel
movements

Volume of feces often increased
Rare blood in feces (melena)
Rare mucus in feces
Tenesmus is uncommon to absent
Concurrent vomiting may be seen

## LARGE INTESTINAL DIARRHEA SIGNS

Weight loss uncommon
Polyphagia rare to absent
Frequency of bowel movements is often greatly
  increased but may be normal
Usually decreased due to increased frequency
Sometimes (hematochezia)
Sometimes mucus in feces
Tenesmus often present
Concurrent vomiting unlikely

## Diseases of the Tongue

### Differential Diagnosis

#### TRAUMA

Mechanical injury (sharp objects)
Chemical injury
Electric shock (electric cord)
Foreign body (plant material, porcupine quill, linear
  foreign bodies)
Sublingual hyperplastic tissue (gum chewer's disease)

#### VIRAL

Calicivirus
Herpesvirus
Papillomavirus

#### NEOPLASIA

Malignant melanoma
Squamous cell carcinoma
Benign tumors (lipoma, plasma cell tumor, granular cell
  tumors, fibroma)

#### METABOLIC DISEASE (UREMIA)

#### SUBLINGUAL MUCOCELE (RANULA)

#### IMMUNE-MEDIATED

Mucous membrane pemphigoid
Pemphigus vulgaris
Bullous pemphigoid
SLE
Autoimmune vasculopathies (idiopathic, infectious, food
  allergies, drug reaction, neoplasia)

**EOSINOPHILIC GRANULOMAS**

**CONTACT MUCOSAL ULCERATION FROM CALCULUS CONTACT**

**CALCINOSIS CIRCUMSCRIPTA**

## Esophageal Disease

### Differential Diagnosis

#### CONGENITAL

Obstruction

Persistent right aortic arch

Persistent right or left subclavian artery

Other vascular ring anomaly

Idiopathic

#### ACQUIRED

Obstruction

Foreign body

Cicatrix/stricture

Neoplasia

- Carcinoma
- *Spirocerca lupi*–induced sarcoma
- Leiomyoma of lower esophageal sphincter
- Extraesophageal neoplasia
  - Thyroid carcinoma
  - Pulmonary carcinoma
  - Mediastinal lymphosarcoma

Achalasia of lower esophageal sphincter (rare)

Gastroesophageal intussusception (rare)

Weakness

Myasthenia (generalized or localized)

Hypoadrenocorticism

Esophagitis

Persistent vomiting

Hiatal hernia

Gastroesophageal reflux/anesthesia-associated reflux

Caustic ingestion (doxycycline, disinfectants, chemicals, etc.)

Foreign body

Excess gastric acidity (gastrinoma, mast cell tumor
[MCT])

Fungal organisms (e.g., pythiosis)

Thermal damage

*Spirocerca lupi* Infection

**Myopathies/Neuropathies**
   Hypothyroidism
   SLE
   Others

**Miscellaneous Causes**
   Lead poisoning
   Chagas disease
   Canine distemper
   Dermatomyositis (principally in Collies)
   Dysautonomia
   Tetanus

**Idiopathic**

## Fecal Incontinence

## Causes

### NONNEUROLOGIC DISEASE

**Colorectal Disease**
   Inflammatory bowel disease
   Neoplasia
   Constipation

**Anorectal Disease**
   Perianal fistula
   Neoplasia
   Surgery (anal sacculectomy, perianal herniorrhaphy,
      rectal resection and anastomosis)

**Miscellaneous**
   Decreased mentation
   Old age
   Severe diarrhea
   Irritable bowel disease

### NEUROLOGIC DISEASE

**Sacral Spinal Cord Disease**
   Discospondylitis
   Neoplasia
   Degenerative myelopathy
   Congenital vertebral malformation
   Sacrococcygeal hypoplasia of Manx cats
   Sacral fracture
   Sacrococcygeal subluxation
   Lumbosacral instability

Lumbosacral nerve root compression
Meningomyelocele
Viral meningomyelitis
Cauda equina syndrome
Vertebral fracture
Fibrocartilaginous embolism

### Peripheral Neuropathy
Trauma
Penetrating wounds
Repair of perineal hernia
Perineal urethrostomy
Hypothyroidism?
Diabetes mellitus?
Dysautonomia

### Central Nervous System
Infectious (distemper, FIP)
Neoplasia
Vascular compromise

## Ileus

## Causes

### PHYSICAL
Intestinal obstruction (foreign body, intussusception, neoplasia, granuloma, torsion, volvulus, incarceration in hernia, adhesions)
Overdistension by aerophagia

### METABOLIC
Uremia
Diabetes mellitus
Hypokalemia
Endotoxemia

### INFLAMMATORY
Parvovirus
Peritonitis
Bacterial enteritis
Other inflammatory causes

### FUNCTIONAL
Abdominal surgery
Peritonitis
Pancreatitis
Ischemia
Irritable bowel syndrome (diarrhea more likely)

**NEUROMUSCULAR**
Anticholinergic drugs
Opioid drugs
Spinal cord injury
Visceral myopathies/neuropathy
Dysautonomia

## Large Intestinal Disease

### Differential Diagnosis

**INFLAMMATION OF LARGE INTESTINE**
Acute colitis/proctitis
Chronic colitis
- Lymphocytic/plasmacytic colitis
- Eosinophilic enterocolitis
- Chronic ulcerative colitis
- Granulomatous colitis (Boxers, French Bulldogs)
Irritable bowel syndrome

**DIETARY INTOLERANCE OR FOOD ALLERGY**

**PARASITES**
Whipworms (*Trichuris* spp.)
*Tritrichomonas* spp. (cats)
Giardiasis
Hookworms (*Ancylostoma* spp.)
*Heterobilharzia americanum*

**BACTERIAL COLITIS**
Clostridial colitis
*Campylobacter* colitis
*Escherichia coli*
*Salmonella* spp.
*Brachyspira pilosicoli*
*Anaerobiospillum* spp. (cats)
*Yersinia enterocolitica*

**FUNGAL COLITIS**
Histoplasmosis
Pythiosis

**VIRAL COLITIS**
FeLV
Infections secondary to FeLV and FIV

### ALGAE (*PROTOTHECA* SPP.)

### PROTOZOA

*Tritrichomonas (Cats)*

### CECOCOLIC INTUSSUSCEPTION

### RECTAL PROLAPSE

### NEOPLASMS OF LARGE INTESTINE

Adenocarcinoma
Lymphoma
Rectal polyps
Leiomyosarcoma

### PYTHIOSIS

### CONSTIPATION

Pelvic canal obstruction caused by malaligned healing of
pelvic fractures
Benign rectal stricture
Dietary indiscretion leading to constipation
Idiopathic megacolon

## Malabsorptive Disease

### Causes

Dietary intolerance or allergy
Parasitism
• Giardiasis
Antibiotic-responsive enteropathy (dysbiosis)
Inflammatory bowel disease
• Lymphocytic/plasmacytic enteritis
• Eosinophilic enteritis
• Idiopathic villous atrophy
• Purulent enteritis
GI lymphoma
Lymphangiectasia
Obstruction caused by neoplasia, infection, or
inflammation
Portal hypertension
Pythiosis
EPI
Cholestatic liver disease/biliary obstruction
Brush border enzyme deficiencies
Brush border transport protein deficiencies
Hyperthyroidism
Gastric hypersecretion
Granulomatous enteritis/gastritis

## Perianal Disease

### Differential Diagnosis

Perineal hernia
Perianal fistulae
Anal sacculitis
Anal sac impaction
Abscessed anal sac
Anal sac (apocrine gland) adenocarcinoma
Perianal gland tumors
- Adenoma (common)
- Adenosarcoma (rare)

## Protein-Losing Enteropathy

### Differential Diagnosis

#### GASTROINTESTINAL HEMORRHAGE
Hemorrhagic gastroenteritis
Ulceration
Neoplasia

#### ENDOPARASITES
*Giardia* spp.
*Ancylostoma* spp.
*Trichuris* spp.
Coccidia
Others

#### INFLAMMATION
Lymphocytic/plasmacytic
Eosinophilic
Granulomatous

#### INFECTION
Parvovirus
Salmonellosis
Histoplasmosis
Phycomycosis

#### STRUCTURAL
Intussusception

#### NEOPLASIA
Lymphosarcoma

#### LYMPHANGIECTASIA
Primary lymphatic disorder
Venous hypertension (e.g., right heart failure)
Hepatic cirrhosis

## Salivary Gland Disease

### Differential Diagnosis

#### SALIVARY NEOPLASIA (MORE COMMON IN CATS THAN DOGS)
Adenocarcinoma
Squamous cell carcinoma
Undifferentiated sarcoma
Mucoepidermoid tumor
Malignant mixed tumor
Sarcoma
Acinic cell carcinoma
Adenoid cystic carcinoma

#### SALIVARY MUCOCELE
Sublingual gland most commonly

#### SIALOADENITIS
Inflammation of the salivary gland

#### SIALOADENOSIS
Noninflammatory, nonneoplastic enlargement of the
salivary gland

## Small Intestinal Disease

### Clinical Findings

Diarrhea
Vomiting
Inappetence/anorexia
Malabsorption
Protein-losing enteropathy
Weight loss
Dehydration
Hematemesis
Melena
Polyphagia
Coprophagia
Abdominal distension
Abdominal pain
Borborygmus/flatulence
Ascites
Edema
Shock
Halitosis
Polydipsia
Ileus
Pica

## Differential Diagnosis

### ACUTE DIARRHEA
Acute enteritis
Dietary indiscretion
Enterotoxemia

### INFECTIOUS DIARRHEA
Canine parvoviral enteritis
Clostridial disease
Feline parvoviral enteritis (panleukopenia)
Canine coronaviral enteritis
Feline coronaviral enteritis
FeLV-associated panleukopenia
FIV-associated diarrhea
Salmon poisoning (*Neorickettsia helminthoeca*)
Campylobacteriosis
Salmonellosis
Histoplasmosis
Miscellaneous bacteria (*Yersinia enterocolitica, Aeromonas hydrophila, Plesiomonas shigelloides*)
Prototheosis (algae)

### ALIMENTARY TRACT PARASITES
Roundworms (*Toxocara* spp.)
Hookworms (*Ancylostoma, Uncinaria* spp.)
Tapeworms (*Dipylidium caninum, Taenia* spp., *Mesocestoides* spp.)
*Strongyloides stercoralis* (in puppies)
Coccidiosis
Cryptosporidia
Giardiasis
Trichomoniasis
Tritrichomoniasis (feline)
*Heterobilharzia*
*Balantidium coli*
*Entamoeba histolytica*

### MALDIGESTIVE DISEASE
EPI

### MALABSORPTIVE DISEASE
Dietary-responsive disease (allergy, intolerance)
Inflammatory bowel disease (lymphocytic/plasmacytic enteritis, canine eosinophilic gastroenteritis)
Feline eosinophilic enteritis/hypereosinophilic syndrome

Granulomatous enteritis
Immunoproliferative enteropathy in Basenjis
Enteropathy in Shar-Peis
Antibiotic-responsive enteropathy

## PROTEIN-LOSING ENTEROPATHY

Intestinal lymphangiectasia
Protein-losing enteropathy in Soft-Coated Wheaten
Terriers

## IRRITABLE BOWEL SYNDROME

## INTESTINAL OBSTRUCTION

Simple intestinal obstruction
Incarcerated intestinal obstruction
Mesenteric torsion/volvulus
Linear foreign object

## INTUSSUSCEPTION

Ileocolic
Jejunojejunal

## SHORT-BOWEL SYNDROME

## NEOPLASIA

Alimentary lymphoma
Intestinal adenocarcinoma
Intestinal leiomyoma/leiomyosarcoma

## Breed Susceptibilities, Dogs

Basenji: lymphocytic/plasmacytic enteritis (immuno-
proliferative disease)
Beagle: cobalamin deficiency
Border Collie: cobalamin deficiency
German Shepherd: idiopathic antibiotic-responsive small
intestinal disease, inflammatory bowel disease (lympho-
plasmacytic, eosinophilic)
Giant Schnauzer: defective cobalamin absorption
Irish Setter: gluten-sensitive enteropathy
Lundehund: lymphangiectasia
Retrievers: dietary allergy
Rottweiler: increased susceptibility to parvoviral enteritis
Soft-Coated Wheaten Terrier: protein-losing enteropathy/
nephropathy
Shar-Pei: lymphocytic/plasmacytic enteritis, cobalamin
deficiency
Yorkshire Terrier: lymphangiectasia
Toy breeds: hemorrhagic gastroenteritis

## Stomach Disorders

## Differential Diagnosis

### GASTRITIS

*Acute Gastritis*

Dietary indiscretion

Dietary intolerance or allergy

Foreign body

Drugs and toxins (NSAIDs, corticosteroids, antibiotics, plants, cleaners, bleach, heavy metals)

Systemic disease (uremia, hepatic disease, hypoadrenocorticism)

Parasites (*Ollulanus* spp., *Physaloptera* spp.)

Bacterial (bacterial toxins, *Helicobacter* spp.)

Viruses

*Hemorrhagic Gastroenteritis*

*Chronic Gastritis*

Lymphocytic/plasmacytic gastritis (inflammatory reaction to a variety of antigens such as *Helicobacter* spp. or *Physaloptera rara*)

Eosinophilic gastritis (allergic reactions to food antigens)

Granulomatous gastritis (e.g., *Ollulanus tricuspis*)

Atrophic gastritis

### GASTRIC OUTFLOW OBSTRUCTION/GASTRIC STASIS

Benign muscular pyloric hypertrophy (pyloric stenosis)

Gastric antral mucosal hypertrophy

Foreign body

Idiopathic gastric hypomotility

Bilious vomiting syndrome

### GASTRIC ULCERATION/EROSION

*Iatrogenic*

NSAIDs

Corticosteroids

NSAID/corticosteroid combinations

*Foreign Body*

*Helicobacter spp*

*Stress Ulceration*

Hypovolemic shock

Septic shock

After gastric dilatation/volvulus

- Neurogenic shock

Hyperacidity
- MCT
- Gastrinoma (rare)

Other causes
- Hepatic disease
- Renal disease
- Hypoadrenocorticism
- Inflammatory disease

*Infiltrative Disease*
Neoplasia
Inflammatory bowel disease
Pythiosis (young dogs, southeastern United States)

## GASTRIC DILATATION/VOLVULUS

## Causes of Acute Abdomen

### GASTROINTESTINAL CAUSES
Acute pancreatitis
Gastroenteritis (parvoviral, bacterial, toxic, hemorrhagic gastroenteritis, etc.)
Gastric dilatation/volvulus
Intestinal obstruction/intussusception/volvulus/ neoplasia
Colitis
Obstipation
Necrosis, rupture, ulceration, or perforation of GI tract
Surgical wound dehiscence
Mesenteric torsion
Duodenocolic ligament entrapment
Pancreatic abscess
Pancreatic neoplasia
Dietary indiscretion
Colonic torsion

### HEPATOBILIARY CAUSES
Acute hepatitis/cholangiohepatitis/leptospirosis/ intoxication
Biliary obstruction
Necrotizing cholecystitis
Hepatic abscess
Bile peritonitis
Liver lobe torsion
Hepatic trauma/rupture
Hepatobiliary neoplasia

### UROGENITAL CAUSES
Urethral or ureteral obstruction/rupture
Pyelonephritis

Renal neoplasia
Acute nephrosis/nephritis
Cystic, renal, ureteral, or urethral calculi
Prostatitis/prostatic abscess/prostatic cyst/prostatic
  neoplasia
Dystocia
Pyometra/uterine rupture
Acute metritis
Renal abscess
Testicular torsion
Ovarian cyst, ovarian neoplasia
Uterine torsion
Uroabdomen
Vaginal rupture

## OTHER CAUSES

Penetrating wound, crush injury
Peritonitis (septic, chemical, urine, bile)
Mesenteric traction (large masses)/lymphadenitis/
  lymphadenopathy/volvulus/avulsion/artery thrombosis
Hemoabdomen (parenchymatous organ rupture)
Neoplasia
Splenic torsion/abscess/mass/rupture
Strangulated hernia
Adhesions with organ entrapment
Pansteatitis
Retroperitoneal hemorrhage
Evisceration
Surgical contamination
Adrenal neoplasia (carcinoma, pheochromocytoma)

## Tonsillar Disorders

### Differential Diagnosis of Tonsillar Disease

Primary viral tonsillitis (bilaterally symmetrical enlarge-
  ment, clinical signs of underlying disease seen such as
  ocular signs, nasal discharge, sneezing)
Primary bacterial tonsillitis (bilaterally symmetrical
  enlargement, may cough if *Bordetella bronchiseptica*, cul-
  ture to confirm)
Secondary tonsillitis (bilaterally symmetrical disease)
- Coughing, vomiting, regurgitation due to concurrent
  disease
- Palate disorder (cleft or elongated)
- Periodontal disease
- Licking at pyoderma or inflamed anal sacs

Foreign body (unilateral enlargement)
- Grass awn
- Splinter
- Bone fragment
- Porcupine quill

Squamous cell carcinoma (unilateral enlargement, biopsy to confirm)

Lymphoma (bilateral enlarged, often other lymphoid organs affected such as lymph nodes or spleen, could biopsy but aspiration of lymph nodes usually easier)

Tonsillar cyst (unilateral enlargement, fluctuant, fluid filled)

# Hematologic Disorders

## Anemia

### Hemolytic Anemia

#### CAUSES/TRIGGERS OF IMMUNE-MEDIATED HEMOLYTIC ANEMIA

*Infection*

Viral

FeLV, FIV, FIP, chronic upper respiratory or GI disease

Bacterial

Leptospirosis, *Mycoplasma haemophilus* infection, salmonellosis, acute and chronic infections (e.g., abscess, pyometra, discospondylitis)

Parasitic

Babesiosis, anaplasmosis, leishmaniasis, dirofilariasis, ehrlichiosis, *Ancylostoma caninum*, *Trichuris vulpis* infection, bartonellosis

*Immune Disorders*

SLE
Hypothyroidism
Primary and secondary immunodeficiencies

*Drugs/Toxins*

Vaccines
Sulfonamides
Methimazole
Procainamide
Cephalosporins
Penicillins
Propylthiouracil
Carprofen

Levamisole
Griseofulvin
Bee-sting envenomation

*Oxidants*
Acetaminophen
Phenothiazines
Vitamin K
Methylene blue
Methionine
Propylene glycol

*Inflammation*
Pancreatitis
Prostatitis/cystitis

*Neoplasia*
Leukemias
Lymphoma
Multiple myeloma
MCT
Splenic hemangioma
Solid tumors (soft tissue sarcomas, bronchoalveolar
carcinoma)

*Genetic Predisposition*
American Cocker Spaniel (most common breed),
English Springer Spaniel, Old English Sheepdog,
Irish Setter, Poodle, Dachshund, Alaskan Malamute,
Schnauzer

## DIFFERENTIATING BLOOD LOSS FROM HEMOLYTIC ANEMIA
*Blood Loss*
Serum or plasma protein concentration
normal-to-low
Clinical evidence of hemorrhage
No icterus, hemoglobinemia, spherocytosis, hemo-
siderinuria, autoagglutination, splenomegaly, or red
blood cell (RBC) changes
Negative direct Coombs test

*Hemolysis*
Serum or plasma protein concentration
normal-to-high
Rarely clinical evidence of hemorrhage
Icterus common
Hemoglobinuria/hemoglobinemia
Spherocytosis
Hemosiderinuria

Autoagglutination sometimes seen
Direct Coombs test usually positive
Splenomegaly
RBC changes numerous

## Nonregenerative Anemia

### DIFFERENTIAL DIAGNOSIS

#### *Anemia of Chronic Disease*

Erythropoietin-Related Conditions
Renal disease
Hypothyroidism
Hypoadrenocorticism
Panhypopituitarism
Growth hormone deficiency
Reduced oxygen requirement
Increased oxygen release

Iron-Deficiency Anemia
Chronic inflammation
Chronic hemorrhage
Dietary iron deficiency

#### *Marrow Disorders*

Toxic Red Cell Aplasia
Estrogen-related
Phenylbutazone-related
Lead poisoning
Other drugs

Hyperestrogenism (ilatrogenic, Neoplastic)

Infection
FeLV
FIV
Parvovirus
Ehrlichiosis
Babesiosis
*Mycoplasma haemofelis*
Endotoxemia

Immunotherapy

Myelofibrosis
FeLV infection
Pyruvate kinase–deficiency anemia
Idiopathic

Myelophthisic Disease
Acute leukemias
Chronic leukemias

Multiple myeloma
Lymphoma
Systemic mast cell disease
Malignant histiocytosis
Metastatic carcinoma
Histoplasmosis

Myelodysplasia
Idiopathic
FeLV/FIV
Preleukemic syndrome

Pure Red Cell Aplasia

*Ineffective Erythropoiesis*
Macrocytic (rare)
Intrinsic marrow disease
Vitamin $B_{12}$ deficiency
Folic acid deficiency

Normocytic

Myelofibrosis
Intrinsic erythroid disease

Microcytic
Iron deficiency
Globin or porphyrin deficiency

Time-Related
Hemolysis or hemorrhage (during the first 3–5 days)

## DIAGNOSIS

*Nonregenerative Anemias Without Other Cytopenias*
Examine bone marrow

Severe Erythroid Hypoplasia
Pure red cell aplasia

Normal-to-Mild Erythroid Hypoplasia
Inflammatory disease
Renal disease
Neoplasia
Hepatic disease
Hypothyroidism
Hypoadrenocorticism

Hypercellular Bone Marrow
Less than 30% blast forms: consider myelodysplastic syndrome
Greater than 30% blast forms: consider hemopoietic neoplasia

*Nonregenerative Anemias With Leukopenia and/or Thrombocytopenia*

Examine bone marrow

Panhypoplasia
Aplastic anemia

Disease Determined by Core Biopsy
Myelonecrosis
Myelofibrosis

Hypercellular Bone Marrow
Less than 30% blast forms: myelodysplastic syndrome
More than 30% blast forms: hemopoietic neoplasia

## Regenerative Anemia

### DIFFERENTIAL DIAGNOSIS

*Hemolysis*

Immune-mediated
- Intravascular
- Extravascular

*Blood Loss Anemia*

Trauma
Coagulopathy
- Clotting factor deficiency
- DIC
- Platelet disorders
- Anticoagulant rodenticides
Endoparasites
GI blood loss
Severe ectoparasites (fleas)

*Oxidative Injury (Heinz Body)*

Onion ingestion
Acetaminophen (cats)
Zinc ingestion (pennies minted after 1982, zinc oxide ointment, zinc-plated bolts and screws)
Benzocaine ingestion (dogs)
DL-Methionine (cats)
Phenolic compounds (mothballs)
Phenazopyridine (cats)

*Erythrocytic Parasites*

Hemotropic *Mycoplasma* spp.
*Babesia* spp.
*Cytauxzoon* spp.

*Fragmentation (Microangiopathic)*
DIC
Heartworm disease
Hemangiosarcoma
Vasculitis
Hemolytic–uremic syndrome
Diabetes mellitus

*Other*
Copper toxicity
Neonatal isoerythrolysis
Hereditary nonspherocytic hemolytic anemia
Pyruvate kinase–deficiency
Feline porphyria
Hemolysis in Abyssinian and Somali cats

## Coagulopathies, Inherited and Acquired

### Differential Diagnosis

#### INHERITED CLOTTING FACTOR DEFICIENCIES

Hemophilia A (factor VIII deficiency), (many breeds, especially German Shepherd, Golden Retriever, domestic shorthair [DSH] cats)

Hemophilia B (factor IX deficiency) (many breeds)

Factor XII deficiency (Hageman trait) (Miniature and Standard Poodles, Shar-Pei, German Shorthaired Pointer, cats)

Vitamin K–dependent factor deficiency: factors II, VII, IX, X (Devon Rex cats)

Factor I: hypofibrinogenemia or dysfibrinogenemia (St. Bernard, Borzoi, Bichon Frise, Collie, DSH cats)

Factor II: hypoprothrombinemia (Boxer, Otterhound, English Cocker Spaniel)

Factor VII: hypoproconvertinemia (Beagle, Malamute, Boxer, Bulldog, Miniature Schnauzer, Scottish Deerhound, DSH cats)

Factor X deficiency (Cocker Spaniel, Parson Russell Terrier, DSH cats)

Hemophilia C (factor XI deficiency: English Springer Spaniel, Great Pyrenees, Kerry Blue Terrier)

Prekallikrein deficiency (Fletcher factor)

#### ACQUIRED CLOTTING FACTOR DEFICIENCY

Liver disease
- Decreased clotting factor production
- Qualitative disorders

Cholestasis
Vitamin K antagonists
Autoimmune disease (lupus anticoagulant)
DIC
Neoplasia

## CLINICAL MANIFESTATIONS OF PRIMARY AND SECONDARY HEMOSTATIC DEFECTS

### *Primary Hemostatic Defects*

Thrombocytopenia and diseases that cause platelet dysfunction such as uremia, von Willebrand disease, monoclonal gammopathies, and vector-borne diseases)—typically see manifestations of superficial bleeding

- Petechiae, ecchymoses
- Bleeding from mucosal surfaces (e.g., bleeding from gingiva, melena, hematochezia, epistaxis, hematuria)
- Bleeding in skin
- Hematomas rare
- Prolonged bleeding immediately after venipuncture

### *Secondary Hemostatic Defects*

Clotting factor deficiencies, rodenticide poisoning, liver disease—typically see manifestations of deep bleeding

- Petechiae, ecchymoses rare
- Hematomas common
- Bleeding into body cavities, joints, muscles
- Delayed bleeding after venipuncture

## Expected Hemostatic Test Results in Selected Diseases

Thrombocytopenia—increased buccal mucosal bleeding time (BMBT), decreased platelet count (PLT), normal activated partial thromboplastin time (aPTT), normal prothrombin time (PT), normal fibrin degradation products (FDP)

Platelet dysfunction (e.g., aspirin treatment)—increased BMBT, normal PLT, increased aPTT, normal PT, normal FDP

Intrinsic pathway defect (e.g., hemophilia A or B)—normal BMBT, normal PLT, increased aPTT, normal PT, normal FDP

Factor VII deficiency—normal BMBT, normal PLT, normal aPTT, increased PT, normal FDP

Multiple factor defects (e.g., vitamin K antagonism)—normal BMBT, normal PLT, increased aPTT, increased PT, normal FDP

Common pathway defect (e.g., factor X deficiency)—normal BMBT, normal PLT, increased aPTT, increased PT, normal FDP

DIC—increased BMBT, decreased PLT, increased aPTT, increased PT, increased FDP

von Willebrand disease—increased BMBT, normal PLT, normal aPTT, normal PT, normal FDP

## Leukocyte Disorders

### Differential Diagnosis

Pelger-Huët anomaly (many breeds of dogs and cats)
- Neutrophil function not altered

Chédiak-Higashi syndrome (blue smoke Persian cats)
- most live a normal lifespan

Canine leukocyte adhesion deficiency: fatal defect (Irish Setters and Irish Setter crosses)

Cyclic hemopoiesis (cyclic neutropenia): fatal defect (gray Collies)

Birman cat neutrophil granulation anomaly: neutrophil function not altered

Hypereosinophilic syndrome (cats): may eventually be fatal

Severe combined immunodeficiency of Parson Russell Terriers: fatal defect

Canine X-linked severe combined immunodeficiency: fatal defect (many breeds)

Defective neutrophil function in Doberman Pinscher: need frequent antimicrobial therapy

Immunodeficiency of Shar-Peis

Immunodeficiency of Weimaraners

Lysosomal storage diseases (many types described, all rare, many breeds)

## Platelet Dysfunction

### Differential Diagnosis

#### ACQUIRED PLATELET DYSFUNCTION

##### Drugs

Prostaglandin inhibitors (NSAIDs)
Vaccines
Antibiotics
Antifungals
Phenothiazines
Aminophylline
Diltiazem

Isoproterenol
Procainamide
Propranolol
Verapamil
Drugs that cause thrombocytopenia
- Cytotoxic drugs (azathioprine, chlorambucil, cyclophosphamide, doxorubicin)
- Miscellaneous (estrogen, methimazole)

*Secondary to Disease*
Renal disease
Liver disease
Myeloproliferative disorders
SLE
Dysproteinemias

*Hereditary*
von Willebrand disease (many breeds)
Canine thrombopathia (Basset Hound, Foxhound, Spitz)
Canine thrombasthenic thrombopathia (Otterhound, Great Pyrenees)
Collagen deficiency diseases/Ehlers-Danlos syndrome (many breeds)

## Splenitis/Splenomegaly

## Differential Diagnosis for Splenomegaly

### SPLENIC MASS (ASYMMETRIC SPLENOMEGALY)
Nodular hyperplasia (lymphoid, fibrohistiocytic)
Hematoma
Neoplasia
- Hemangiosarcoma
- Hemangioma
- Leiomyosarcoma
- Fibrosarcoma
- Histiocytic sarcoma
- Leiomyoma
- Myelolipoma
- Metastatic disease

Abscess
Extramedullary hematopoiesis
Granuloma

### UNIFORM SPLENOMEGALY
*Congestion*
Drugs
Portal hypertension

Right-sided heart failure
Splenic torsion

*Hyperplasia*
Chronic infection
Inflammatory bowel disease
SLE
Polycythemia vera

*Extramedullary Hematopoiesis*
Chronic anemia
Immune-mediated hemolytic anemia
Immune-mediated thrombocytopenia

*Neoplasia*
Lymphoma
Systemic mastocytosis
Primary MCT
Metastatic neoplasia
Multiple myeloma
Acute and chronic leukemias
Malignant histiocytosis
Polycythemia vera

*Nonneoplastic Infiltrative Disease*
Amyloidosis
Hypereosinophilic syndrome (cats)

*Inflammation*
Suppurative
Sepsis
Bacterial endocarditis
Infectious canine hepatitis
Foreign body
Penetrating wounds
Toxoplasmosis

*Granulomatous*
Cryptococcosis
Histoplasmosis
Mycobacteriosis
Leishmaniasis

*Pyogranulomatous*
FIP
Blastomycosis
Sporotrichosis

*Eosinophilic*
Eosinophilic gastroenteritis
Hypereosinophilic syndrome
Neoplasia

*Lymphoplasmacytic*

Ehrlichiosis
Hemotropic mycoplasmosis
Lymphoplasmacytic enteritis
Pyometra
Brucellosis
Anaplasmosis

*Necrotic Tissue*

Torsion
Necrotic center of neoplasms
Infectious canine hepatitis
Anaerobic infection
Systemic calicivirosis
Tularemia
Salmonellosis

## Infectious Causes

### VIRAL

FeLV
FIV
FIP
Infectious canine hepatitis

### BACTERIAL

Canine brucellosis
Mycoplasmosis
Borreliosis
Plague
Tularemia
Streptococcosis
Staphylococcosis
Salmonellosis
*Francisella* infection
Endotoxemia

### FUNGAL

Cryptococcosis
Histoplasmosis
Blastomycosis

### RICKETTSIAL

Ehrlichiosis
Rocky Mountain spotted fever
Q fever (*Coxiella burnetii*)
*Mycoplasma haemofelis*

### PROTOZOAL

Toxoplasmosis
Cytauxzoonosis (cat)

Babesiosis (*Babesia canis* and *B. gibsoni*)
Leishmaniasis (dog)

## Thrombocytopenia

## Differential Diagnosis

### INCREASED PLATELET DESTRUCTION/SEQUESTRATION/UTILIZATION
Immune-mediated thrombocytopenia
Drug-induced thrombocytopenia
Infectious (*Anaplasma* spp., *Bartonella* spp., sepsis)
Microangiopathy
DIC
Neoplasia (immune-mediated, microangiography)
Live viral vaccine–induced thrombocytopenia
Hemolytic–uremic syndrome/thrombotic thrombocytopenic purpura
Vasculitis
Splenomegaly
Splenic torsion
Endotoxemia
Acute hepatic necrosis
Hemorrhage

### DECREASED PLATELET PRODUCTION
Drug-induced megakaryocytic hypoplasia (estrogen, phenylbutazone, melphalan, lomustine, beta-lactams)
Myelophthisis
Idiopathic bone marrow aplasia
Retroviral infection (FeLV/FIV)
Immune-mediated megakaryocytic hypoplasia
Cyclic thrombocytopenia
Idiopathic bone marrow aplasia
Ehrlichiosis

# Immunologic and Immune-Mediated Disorders

## Autoimmune Skin Diseases

### Differential Diagnosis

#### GENERALIZED PUSTULAR/CRUSTING DERMATOSIS

Pemphigus foliaceus (PF) (nose, ear pinna, and footpad typically affected)

Superficial pustular drug reactions (nasal and footpad lesions may be absent)

Others: rare presentation—SLE, sterile eosinophilic pustulosis, linear immunoglobulin A (IgA) pustular dermatosis, subcorneal pustular dermatosis

#### FOCAL PUSTULAR/CRUSTING DERMATOSIS

Face, footpads: PF

Face and ears only: PF (early), pemphigus erythematosus (PE), drug eruptions, lupus erythematosus

Nasal only: DLE, PF (early), PE

#### MUCOCUTANEOUS AND MUCOSAL ULCERATIONS

Pemphigus vulgaris (may also have oral lesions)

Mucous membrane bullous pemphigoid

Epidermolysis bullosa acquisita

EM (target lesions, cutaneous lesions)

Bullous SLE

Drug reactions

Linear IgA bullous dermatosis, toxic epidermal necrolysis (rare)

#### NONMUCOSAL ULCERATIONS (AXILLAE, INGUINAE, PINNAE, OTHER HAIRY AREAS)

Bullous pemphigoid

Epidermolysis bullosa acquisita

Linear IgA bullous dermatosis

Bullous SLE

Canine vesicular cutaneous lupus erythematosus
  (idiopathic ulcerative dermatosis of Collies, Shetland
  Sheepdogs)

EM

Toxic epidermal necrolysis

Drug eruptions

Pemphigus vulgaris

### DEPIGMENTING SKIN DISEASES

Nasal only: DLE, vitiligo-like syndrome, uveodermatologic syndrome, early PF or PE

Nose, footpad, lip, eyelid, mucocutaneous area: uveodermatologic syndrome (uveitis also)

Hair coat or skin: idiopathic leukotrichia or leukoderma

### MISCELLANEOUS

Focal alopecia: alopecia areata, rabies vaccine, focal
  vasculitis

Widespread noninflammatory alopecia: alopecia areata,
  pseudopelade

Erythematous target lesions: EM

Nodular ulcerative lesions: nodular panniculitis

Purpura, hemorrhage, punched-out lesions

Ear margin necrosis, dependent edema: vasculitis, proliferative necrotizing otitis of kittens, cryoglobulinemia
  and cryofibrinogenemia, proliferative thrombovascular
  necrosis of the pinnae

Scaling, follicular casts, alopecia: sebaceous adenitis

Claw and claw bed disease: symmetric lupoid
  onychodystrophy

## Immune-Mediated Disease

## Laboratory Diagnosis

### DIRECT COOMBS TEST

Immune-mediated hemolytic anemia

Hemolytic anemia in SLE

### SLIDE AGGLUTINATION TEST

Immune-mediated hemolytic anemia

### ANTIPLATELET ANTIBODIES

Immune-mediated thrombocytopenia

### ANTINEUTROPHIL ANTIBODIES

Immune-mediated neutropenia

### THYROXIN AND THYROGLOBULIN AUTOANTIBODIES
Hypothyroidism

### ACETYLCHOLINE RECEPTOR AUTOANTIBODIES
Myasthenia gravis

### C-REACTIVE PROTEIN
Nonspecific biochemical marker of inflammation, may be useful for monitoring treatment response

### 2M MYOFIBER AUTOANTIBODIES
Masticatory muscle myositis

### ANTINUCLEAR ANTIBODY
SLE
Chronic antigenic stimulation

### RHEUMATOID FACTOR
Rheumatoid arthritis (RA)

### DIRECT IMMUNOFLUORESCENCE
Antibody-complement deposition

### IMMUNOHISTOCHEMISTRY
Detect presence of antibody in fixed tissues

## Differential Diagnosis for Immune-Mediated Arthritis

### EROSIVE IMMUNE-MEDIATED ARTHRITIDES
RA (dog, rarely in cat)
Periosteal proliferative polyarthritis (cat, rarely in dog)

### NONEROSIVE IMMUNE-MEDIATED ARTHRITIDES
Idiopathic polyarthritis
- **Type I:** uncomplicated idiopathic arthritis (most common)
- **Type II:** idiopathic arthritis associated with infection remote from joints—respiratory tract, tonsils, conjunctiva (chlamydia in cats), urinary tract, uterus, skin, oral cavity
- **Type III:** idiopathic arthritis associated with gastroenteritis
- **Type IV:** idiopathic arthritis associated with malignant neoplasia—squamous cell carcinoma, heart base tumor, leiomyoma, mammary carcinoma, myeloproliferative disease (cats)

SLE
Drug-induced polyarthritis

- Sulfas, lincomycin, erythromycin, cephalosporins, penicillins, trimethoprim-sulfa (especially Doberman Pinscher)

Vaccination reaction

Polyarthritis/polymyositis syndrome

Polyarthritis/meningitis syndrome

Familial renal amyloidosis in Chinese Shar-Peis

Polyarthritis in adolescent Akitas

Polyarthritis nodosa (inflammatory condition of small arteries—histopathologic diagnosis)

## Immune System Components

### Function

#### HUMORAL IMMUNITY

*B Lymphocytes and Plasma Cells*
Production of immunoglobulins

#### CELLULAR IMMUNITY

*T Lymphocytes*
Production of lymphokines
Helper T cells
- Stimulate immune reactivity
Suppressor T cells
- Suppress immune reactivity
Antibody-dependent, cell-mediated cytotoxicity
Natural killer cells
- Direct cytotoxicity

#### PHAGOCYTIC CELLS

*Mononuclear Phagocytic Cells*
Antigen presentation
Phagocytosis of particles

*Neutrophils and Eosinophils*
Phagocytosis of particles
Antibody-dependent, cell-mediated cytotoxicity

## Mechanisms of Immunopathologic Injury

### Type I (Immediate)

Humoral immune system (T-helper cells and B cells), IgE, mast cells, inflammatory mediators

Skin, respiratory tract, GI tract commonly affected

Examples include acute anaphylactic reaction, atopy, allergic bronchitis, feline asthma

## Type II (Cytotoxic)

Humoral immune system (IgG and IgM)

Hematologic systems, neuromuscular junctions, and skin commonly affected

Examples include immune-mediated hemolytic anemia, immune-mediated thrombocytopenia, myasthenia gravis, PF

## Type III (Immune Complex)

Soluble immune complexes

Kidney, joints, and skin commonly affected

Examples include glomerulonephritis, SLE, RA

## Type IV (Delayed Type)

Sensitized T lymphocytes, cytokines, neutrophils, and macrophages

Endocrine glands, muscle commonly affected

Examples include lymphocytic thyroiditis, myositis

## Organ Systems Affected by Autoimmune Disorders in the Dog and Cat

### Differential Diagnosis

#### HEMATOLOGIC

Immune-mediated hemolytic anemia

Pure red cell aplasia

Immune-mediated thrombocytopenia

Idiopathic neutropenia

#### JOINTS

See Differential Diagnosis for Immune-Mediated Arthritis

#### SKIN

See Autoimmune Skin Diseases

#### EYE

Uveitis

Retinitis

Pannus

#### KIDNEY

Glomerulonephritis

#### RESPIRATORY TRACT

Allergic rhinitis

Allergic bronchitis (asthma)

Pulmonary infiltrates with eosinophils

### GASTROINTESTINAL TRACT
Feline stomatitis, gingivitis
Lymphocytic, plasmacytic enteritis
Anal furunculosis (perianal fistula)

### NEUROLOGIC SYSTEM
Myasthenia gravis
Myositis
Polyradiculoneuritis
Granulomatous meningoencephalitis
Polyarteritis

### ENDOCRINE GLANDS
Thyroiditis (hypothyroidism)
Adrenalitis (hypoadrenocorticism)
Insulitis (diabetes mellitus)

### MULTISYSTEMIC IMMUNE DISEASE
SLE

## Systemic Lupus Erythematosus

### Organs and Tissues Affected

RBCs
- Immune-mediated hemolytic anemia
- Pure red cell aplasia

Platelets
- Immune-mediated thrombocytopenia

Glomeruli
- Glomerulonephritis

Synovium
- Nonerosive polyarthritis

Blood vessels
- Vasculitis

Epidermis
- Dermatitis

Neutrophils
- Immune-mediated neutrophilia

Clotting factors
- Coagulopathy

Central nervous system
- Seizures, focal signs

Skeletal muscle/nerve end plate
- Polymyositis
- Polyneuritis
- Myasthenia gravis

## Criteria for Diagnosis in Dogs and Cats

SLE is diagnosed when three or more of the following criteria are manifested simultaneously or at any time: antinuclear antibodies (ANAs)

- Abnormal ANA titer in the absence of drugs or infectious or neoplastic conditions known to be associated with abnormal titers

Cutaneous lesions

- Depigmentation, erythema, erosions, ulcerations, crusts, scaling, with biopsy findings consistent with SLE

Oral ulcers

- Oral or nasopharyngeal ulceration, usually painless

Arthritis

- Nonerosive, nonseptic arthritis involving two or more peripheral joints

Renal disorders

- Glomerulonephritis or persistent proteinuria in the absence of UTI

Anemia/thrombocytopenia

- Hemolytic anemia/thrombocytopenia in the absence of offending drugs

Leukopenia

- Low total white cell count

Polymyositis or myocarditis

- Inflammatory disease of skeletal or cardiac muscles

Serositis

- Presence of a nonseptic inflammatory cavity effusion (abdominal, pleural, or pericardial)

Neurologic disorders

- Seizures or psychosis in the absence of known disorders

Antiphospholipids

- Prolongation of aPTT that fails to correct with a 1:1 mixture of patient's and normal plasma, in the absence of heparin or FDPs

# SECTION VII

# Infectious Disease

## Anaplasmosis, Canine

### Clinical Signs

Infection may be subclinical
Fever
Depression
Inappetence
Scleral injection
Lameness, stiffness, reluctance to move
Coughing (soft and nonproductive)
Lymphadenopathy
Splenomegaly
Neutrophilic polyarthritis (rare)
Central nervous system (CNS) signs?
Vomiting/diarrhea
May be more susceptible to other infections

#### LABORATORY ABNORMALITIES

Thrombocytopenia
Lymphopenia
Eosinopenia
Mild regenerative anemia
Hypoalbuminemia
Mild to moderately elevated hepatic enzymes

## Bacterial Infections, Systemic

## Differential Diagnosis

### LEPTOSPIROSIS

Hepatic dysfunction, renal dysfunction, fever, anterior uveitis, icterus

Coagulation abnormalities, vomiting/diarrhea, icterus, polyuria/polydipsia, anorexia

Some cases may be subclinical

### BORRELIOSIS (LYME DISEASE)

Fever, inappetence/lethargy, lymphadenopathy, polyarthritis

Glomerulonephritis/acute, progressive renal failure, mild dermatologic lesions

Meningitis/encephalitis (rare), myocarditis

### MYCOBACTERIOSIS

Often asymptomatic, skin lesions, dermal nodules, draining tracts, lymphadenopathy, bronchopneumonia, pulmonary nodules, hilar lymphadenopathy, vomiting, diarrhea secondary to intestinal malabsorption, feline leprosy

### BRUCELLOSIS (DOGS)

Clinical signs may be mild to absent

Fever, lymphadenopathy

Epididymitis, scrotal enlargement, scrotal dermatitis, infertility in males

Abortion, early embryonic death, fetal resorption, in pregnant bitches

Discospondylitis

Rarely uveitis, glomerulonephritis, meningoencephalitis

### TETANUS

Localized tetanus, especially cats; stiffness in a muscle of limb

Generalized tetanus stiff gait, outstretched or dorsally curved tails, extreme muscle rigidity, hypersensitivity to touch, light, and sounds

Ears erect, lips drawn back (sardonic grin), protrusion of globe, enophthalmos

Trismus (lockjaw), laryngeal spasm, regurgitation, megaesophagus leading to aspiration pneumonia, seizures

### BOTULISM

Generalized lower motor neuron and parasympathetic dysfunction, CN signs, mentation is normal

Quadriplegia, megaesophagus, respiratory paralysis; may lead to death

### FELINE PLAGUE (*YERSINIA PESTIS*)
Spread by fleas
May show signs of bubonic, septicemic, and pneumonic plague
Depression
Cervical swellings, draining tracts
Dyspnea or cough

### MYCOPLASMOSIS/UREAPLASMOSIS (CATS)
Conjunctivitis, sneezing, mucopurulent nasal discharge, coughing, dyspnea, fever, lameness, swollen joints, subcutaneous abscessation

## Members of the Order Rickettsiales of Clinical Importance in Dogs and Cats

### RICKETTSIOSES (SPOTTED FEVER GROUP RICKETTSIAE)
*Rickettsia rickettsia*
Species of the following tick genera transmit spotted fever group agents: *Dermacentor*, *Rhipicephalus*, *Haemaphysalis*, and *Amblyomma*

### EHRLICHIOSIS (CANINE)
*Ehrlichia canis, E. chaffeensis, E. ewingii, E. muris*, and *E. ruminantium*

### ANAPLASMOSIS (CANINE AND FELINE)
*Anaplasma phagocytophilum*
*Anaplasma platys* (canine cyclic thrombocytopenia: mildly pathogenic)

### NEORICKETTSIOSIS
*Neorickettsia helminthoeca, N. risticii*

### BARTONELLOSIS, CANINE
*Clinical Findings*
Many species of *Bartonella* are suspected to cause disease in dogs (e.g., *B. vinsonii, B. henselae, B. clarridgeiae, B. elizabethae*)
Fever
Endocarditis, myocarditis, arrhythmias
Thromboembolic disease
Epistaxis
Intermittent lameness
Bone pain
Granulomatous lymphadenitis
Dermatologic lesions/cutaneous vasculitis/panniculitis
Anterior uveitis
Polyarthritis

Meningoencephalitis
Immune-mediated hemolytic anemia
Immune-mediated thrombocytopenia
Eosinophilia
Peliosis hepatitis
Hemangiopericytoma
Bacillary angiomatosis
Granulomatous hepatitis
Chronic weight loss
Hyperviscosity syndrome

## BARTONELLOSIS, FELINE
### *Subclinical Disease in Most Cats*
Uveitis?
Endocarditis?

Anaplasmosis
*Anaplasma phagocytophilum*, formally known as
*Ehrlichia equi, E. phagocytophila*

Cause of Canine Granulocytic Ehrlichiosis
Clinical signs
- Fever
- Depression
- Inappetence
- Scleral injection
- Lameness/polyarthritis
- Hemorrhage, epistaxis, melena, petechiae
- Coughing
- Lymphadenopathy
- Splenomegaly
- Vomiting/diarrhea
- Lymphopenia, eosinopenia, mild nonregenerative anemia
- Hypoalbuminemia, elevated hepatic enzymes
- Proprioceptive deficits or other signs of meningitis

## ANAPLASMA PLATYS
### *Cause of Canine Thrombocytic Anaplasmosis*
Forms of Morula That Can Be Visualized in Platelets
Clinical signs:
- Majority of cases in United States have been mild or subclinical
More severe signs in European or South American cases include:
- Fever
- Splenomegaly
- Hemorrhage

## Ehrlichiosis, Canine

### Clinical Findings

#### ACUTE
Fever
Anorexia/weight loss
Depression
Serous or purulent oculonasal discharge
Lymphadenopathy/splenomegaly
Peripheral edema
Petechial and ecchymotic hemorrhages
Neurologic signs (ataxia, seizures, vestibular signs,
   hyperesthesia, CN defects)
Dyspnea
History of recent or present tick bite
Thrombocytopenia
Leukopenia followed by leukocytosis and monocytosis
Low-grade nonregenerative anemia, unless hemorrhage
Variable *Ehrlichia* titer, PCR positive

#### SUBCLINICAL
No clinical abnormalities apparent
Hyperglobulinemia, thrombocytopenia, neutropenia,
   lymphocytosis, monocytosis
Positive *Ehrlichia* titer, PCR positive

#### CHRONIC
Depression
Pale mucous membranes
Weight loss
Abdominal pain
Splenomegaly
Epistaxis, retinal hemorrhage, petechia and ecchymoses,
   melena, hematochezia, hematuria, and other examples
   of hemorrhage
Lymphadenopathy
Stiffness, swollen/painful joints, polymyositis
Hepatomegaly
Dyspnea, interstitial or alveolar lung infiltrates
Perivascular retinitis, hyphema, retinal detachment,
   anterior uveitis, corneal edema
Seizures, paresis, meningeal pain, CN deficits
Arrhythmias
Polyuria/polydipsia
Secondary opportunistic infection (viral papillomatosis,
   protozoal infections, bacteriuria)

Monocytosis, lymphocytosis, thrombocytopenia, nonregenerative anemia, hyperglobulinemia, hypoalbuminemia, hypocellular bone marrow, proteinuria, polyclonal or monoclonal gammopathy, nonseptic suppurative polyarthritis, cerebrospinal fluid (CSF) mononuclear pleocytosis

Increased ALT and ALP

Positive *Ehrlichia* titer, PCR positive

## Influenza, Canine

### Clinical Features

**H3N8 strain**—originated in Florida, thought to have mutated from equine flu strain; most outbreaks in group housed dogs (racetracks, animal shelters).

**H3N2 strain**—outbreak in 2015 started in Chicago. Thought to have resulted from direct transfer of avian influenza virus in markets in Asia (Korea, Thailand, China).

Individual pets often had a recent history of exposure to other dogs.

Mild form may cause a harsh cough similar to cough heard with infectious tracheobronchitis.

More commonly, cough is soft and moist, cough may persist for as long as a month.

Fever (may reach 104–106°F with severe form).

Mucopurulent nasal discharge.

Increased respiratory rate progressing to respiratory distress.

May progress to overt pneumonia (severe form).

Mortality rate less than 5%. Very young and very old are most at risk.

## Influenza, Feline

Transition of H3N2, H1N1, H3N8, H5N2, H9N2, HFN1 causing mild disease in cats has been documented.

In late 2016, over 40 cats tested positive for a low pathogenic avian influenza virus A, H7N2, in a shelter in Manhattan, New York.

## Mycoses, Systemic

### Clinical Findings

#### BLASTOMYCOSIS *(BLASTOMYCES DERMATITIDIS)*

Restricted primarily to Mississippi, Ohio, Missouri, Tennessee, and St. Lawrence River valleys plus the southern Great Lakes and the southern Mid-Atlantic states. Recent reports of cases in northern California and Pacific Northwest. Also seen in Canada (Alberta,

Manitoba, Ontario, Quebec, Saskatchewan), Central America, and Africa.

Sporting breeds predisposed because of greater exposure, males more than females

Anorexia, depression, weight loss, cachexia, fever, mild-to-severe dyspnea, cyanosis, cough, chylothorax, diffuse lymphadenopathy, papules, plaques and ulcerative nodules, paronychia, chorioretinitis, conjunctivitis, keratitis, iridocyclitis, anterior uveitis, subretinal granulomas, retinal detachment, secondary glaucoma, lameness from osteomyelitis, splenomegaly

Radiographically, infiltrative bronchointerstitial and alveolar disease, hilar lymphadenopathy

## HISTOPLASMOSIS *(HISTOPLASMA CAPSULATUM)*

Restricted primarily to Mississippi, Missouri, and Ohio River valleys and Mid-Atlantic states

Sporting breeds predisposed because of greater exposure

Common clinical signs include anorexia, fever, depression, weight loss, cough, dyspnea, diarrhea (large bowel diarrhea most often, may see protein-losing enteropathy), hepatosplenomegaly, icterus, ascites, and lymphadenopathy.

Less common signs include lameness secondary to osteomyelitis or polyarthritis, chorioretinitis, CNS disease, and cutaneous lesions.

### *Differential Diagnosis for Gastrointestinal Signs Seen in Dogs and Cats With Histoplasmosis*

Large Intestinal Disease

Diet-associated colitis
- Dietary hypersensitivity
- Foreign material–induced colitis

Idiopathic colitis
- Lymphocytic–plasmacytic colitis
- Eosinophilic colitis
- Granulomatous colitis
- Histiocytic ulcerative colitis of Boxers dogs
- Suppurative colitis

Parasitic and protozoal colitis
- Trichuriasis (whipworm)
- Ancylostomiasis (hookworm)
- Entamebiasis
- Balantidiasis
- Giardiasis

Bacterial colitis
- Salmonellosis
- *Campylobacter jejuni*
- *Yersinia enterocolitica, Y. pseudotuberculosis*
- Mycobacteria
- *Clostridium perfringens, C. difficile*

Fungal colitis
- *Candidiasis*
- GI pythiosis
- Protothecosis

Cecocolic or ileocolic intussusception

Pancreatitis-associated colitis

### Small Intestinal Disease

Idiopathic inflammatory bowel disease
- Lymphocytic–plasmacytic enteritis
- Eosinophilic enteritis
- Granulomatous enteritis

Intestinal lymphosarcoma

Parasitic enteritis
- Ancylostomiasis
- Toxocariasis
- Chronic giardiasis

Infectious enteritis
- Small intestinal bacterial overgrowth
- GI pythiosis

Lymphangiectasia

EPI

Partial intestinal obstruction

Chronic enteropathy of Shar-Peis

Immunoproliferative enteritis of Basenjis

## COCCIDIOIDOMYCOSIS *(COCCIDIOIDES IMMITIS, COCCIDIOIDES POSADASII)*

Primarily southwestern United States, California, Mexico, Central and South America

Common clinical signs include lameness with swollen and painful joints and bones, cough, dyspnea, anorexia, weakness, pleural effusion, and cutaneous lesions over infected bones

Less common signs include myocarditis, icterus, renomegaly, splenomegaly, hepatomegaly, orchitis, epididymitis, keratitis, iritis, granulomatous uveitis, glaucoma, seizures, ataxia, and central vestibular disease

## CRYPTOCOCCOSIS *(CRYPTOCOCCUS NEOFORMANS, CRYPTOCOCCUS GATTII)*

Found worldwide, more common in southern United States, most common in cats

*C. gattii* found in subtropics, British Columbia, and United States Pacific Northwest

Common clinical signs include upper respiratory signs, unilateral-to-bilateral nasal discharge, soft masses in nasal cavity or over bridge of nose, ulcerative skin lesions, lymphadenopathy, granulomatous chorioretinitis, and retinal detachment

Less common signs include fever, lung involvement, CNS involvement caused by invasion through cribriform plate, depression, seizures, circling, ataxia, blindness, head pressing, and paresis

## ASPERGILLOSIS (*ASPERGILLUS* SPP.)

Dogs affected more often than cats, German Shepherd dogs overrepresented

Nasal turbinate destruction, frontal sinus osteomyelitis, mucoid to hemorrhagic nasal discharge, epistaxis

May lead to masticatory muscle atrophy and CNS disease by erosion through cribriform plate

In rare cases, disseminates and causes multiple organ disease

## PYTHIOSIS, LAGENIDIOSIS *(PYTHIUM INSIDIOSUM, LAGENIDIUM GIGANTEUM)*

Severe, often fatal, chronic GI and cutaneous diseases

## ZYGOMYCOSIS (MULTIPLE FUNGI IN CLASS ZYGOMYCETES)

Nasopharyngeal involvement, poorly responsive to therapy

## Differential Diagnosis for Systemic Manifestations

Multisystemic granulomatous, neoplastic, and immune-mediated diseases must be differentiated from disseminated systemic mycoses

### DIFFERENTIAL DIAGNOSIS FOR NODULAR SKIN DISEASE

*Bacteria Skin Disease*

Actinomycosis

Mycobacteriosis

Botryomycosis

Brucellosis

*Rhodococcus equi* infection

*Bartonella vinsonii* subsp. *berkhoffi* infection

*Mycotic and Miscellaneous Infectious Skin Disease*
  Cryptococcosis
  Blastomycosis
  Coccidioidomycosis
  Sporotrichosis
  Basidiobolomycosis
  Conidiobolomycosis
  Phaeohyphomycosis
  Hyalohyphomycosis
  Eumycotic mycetoma
  Dermatophytic mycetoma
  Prototothecosis
  Pythiosis
  Lagenidiosis
  Nodular leishmaniasis

*Noninfectious Pyogranulomatous Skin Disease*
  Foreign body reaction
  Idiopathic nodular panniculitis
  Sebaceous adenitis (nodular form)
  Canine cutaneous sterile pyogranulomatous/granu-
    loma syndrome

*Neoplasia*
  Squamous cell carcinoma
  Cutaneous lymphoma
  Mycosis fungoides (cutaneous T-cell lymphoma)
  Cutaneous histiocytosis

*Miscellaneous Diseases*
  SLE
  Systemic vasculitis
  Cutaneous embolic disease

# Differential Diagnosis for Chorioretinitis, Exudative Retinal Detachment, and Panophthalmitis

## FUNGAL
  Blastomycosis
  Cryptococcosis
  Coccidioidomycosis
  Geotrichosis
  Histoplasmosis
  Aspergillosis

## NEOPLASIA
  Lymphosarcoma
  Metastatic neoplasia

## MISCELLANEOUS INFECTIOUS CAUSES

Prototothecosis

Brucellosis

Toxoplasmosis

*Neospora caninum* infection

Leishmaniasis

Lymphadenopathy must be differentiated from numerous causes, including lymphosarcoma, other fungal infections, rickettsial diseases, brucellosis, mycobacteriosis, prototothecosis, and leishmaniasis

Solitary bone lesions must be differentiated from primary or metastatic neoplasia and other fungal or bacterial osteomyelitis

## Neorickettsiosis, Canine

### *Neorickettsia helminthoeca* (Salmon Poisoning Disease)

Restricted to western slopes of Cascade Mountains from northern California to southern Vancouver Island

Vector is a fluke—*Nanophyetus salmincola;* dogs become infected from ingesting parasitized fish

#### CLINICAL SIGNS

Fever

Anorexia/weight loss

Depression

Lymphadenopathy

Vomiting

Diarrhea

Hematochezia

Neutrophilia with left shift, lymphopenia, monocytosis, thrombocytopenia

Electrolyte derangements, elevated hepatic enzymes, hypoalbuminemia

### *Neorickettsia risticii*

Cause of equine Potomac horse fever

Vector is suspected to be a fluke—*Acanthatrium oregonense*

Has been identified by culture and PCR in dogs with the following signs

#### CLINICAL SIGNS

Lethargy

Intermittent vomiting

Bleeding tendencies

Polyarthritis

Neurologic signs
Dependent edema
Anemia
Thrombocytopenia

## Polysystemic Protozoal Diseases

### Clinical Findings

#### FELINE TOXOPLASMOSIS (*TOXOPLASMA GONDII*)

Acute toxoplasmosis: may induce a self-limiting, small
bowel diarrhea

Disseminated toxoplasmosis: overwhelming intracellular
replication of tachyzoites after primary infection—
depression, anorexia, fever, hypothermia, peritoneal
effusion, icterus, dyspnea, death—coinfection with
FeLV, FIV, FIP, and others may predispose to disseminated toxoplasmosis

Chronic toxoplasmosis: anterior or posterior uveitis,
fever, muscle hyperesthesia, weight loss, anorexia,
seizures, ataxia, icterus, diarrhea, pancreatitis

#### CANINE TOXOPLASMOSIS (*TOXOPLASMA GONDII*)

Respiratory, GI, neuromuscular signs: fever, vomiting,
diarrhea, dyspnea, icterus, ataxia, seizures, tremors,
CN deficits, paresis, paralysis, myositis, lower motor
neuron disease, myocardial disease, chorioretinitis,
anterior uveitis, iridocyclitis, optic neuritis (ocular
lesions less common in dogs than cats)

#### NEOSPOROSIS (*NEOSPORA CANINUM*)

Most common in neonates but can be seen at any age

Ascending paralysis, hyperextension of hind limbs,
muscle atrophy, polymyositis, multifocal CNS disease,
myocarditis, dysphagia, ulcerative dermatitis, pneumonia, hepatitis

#### BABESIOSIS (*BABESIA CANIS, BABESIA GIBSONI*)

Anemia, fever, pale mucous membranes, tachycardia,
tachypnea, depression, anorexia, weakness, icterus,
petechiae, hepatosplenomegaly, DIC, metabolic acidosis, renal disease

#### CYTAUXZOONOSIS (*CYTAUXZOONOSIS FELIS*)

Only in domestic and wild cats

Fever, anorexia, dyspnea (pneumonitis), depression,
icterus, pale mucous membranes, death

## HEPATOZOONOSIS *(HEPATOZOON CANIS, H. AMERICANUM)*

Most common in puppies and immunosuppressed dogs, but *H. americanum* can be primary

Fever, weight loss, severe hyperesthesia, anorexia, anemia, depression, oculonasal discharge, bloody diarrhea

## LEISHMANIASIS *(LEISHMANIA INFANTUM, LEISHMANIA BRAZILIENSIS* IN SOUTH AMERICA, *LEISHMANIA TROPICA,* AND *L. MAJOR* IN ASIA AND NORTH AFRICA)

Weight loss, normal-to-increased appetite, polyuria/polydipsia, muscle wasting, depression, vomiting, diarrhea, cough, epistaxis, sneezing, melena, splenomegaly, facial alopecia, rhinitis, dermatitis, icterus, swollen and painful joints, uveitis, conjunctivitis

Dermatologic lesions include hyperkeratosis, scaling, mucocutaneous ulcers, and intradermal nodules on muzzle, ears, and footpads.

## AMERICAN TRYPANOSOMIASIS *(TRYPANOSOMA CRUZI)*

Acute infection: myocarditis, heart failure—lymphadenopathy, pale mucous membranes, tachycardia, pulse deficits, hepatomegaly, abdominal distension, anorexia, diarrhea, neurologic signs

Chronic infection: those that survive acute infection may present with chronic dilative cardiomyopathy—right-sided heart failure, conductive disturbances, supraventricular arrhythmias

## Rocky Mountain Spotted Fever

### Clinical Findings

Depression/lethargy
Fever
Anorexia
Myalgia/arthralgia
Lymphadenopathy
Vestibular deficits
Conjunctivitis/scleral congestion/hyphema/iridal and retinal hemorrhage
Pneumonitis/dyspnea/cough
Abdominal pain
Edema of face and extremities
Epistaxis
Melena
Hematuria
Anterior uveitis
Rash/petechiae

Nausea/vomiting
Diarrhea
Vasculitis/thrombocytopenia/DIC
Hyperesthesia/spinal cord signs
Seizures
Cardiac arrhythmias
Icterus
Acute renal failure
Coma/stupor
Polyuria/polydipsia

## Sepsis and Systemic Inflammatory Response Syndrome (SIRS)

### Definitions

*Bacteremia:* the presence of viable bacteria in the bloodstream

*Sepsis:* infection-induced systemic inflammation

*Severe sepsis:* organ dysfunction and manifestations of hypoperfusion or hypotension secondary to sepsis

*Septic shock:* hypotension secondary to sepsis, not responsive to intravenous (IV) fluid therapy

*SIRS:* systemic inflammation caused by either infectious or noninfectious processes; diagnosis based on fulfillment of at least two of four criteria (tachycardia, tachypnea, hypothermia, or hyperthermia and either leukocytosis, leucopenia, or bands)

*Multiple organ dysfunction syndrome (MODS):* altered function of two or more organs secondary to SIRS such that homeostasis cannot be maintained without intervention

*Acute respiratory distress syndrome:* a pulmonary inflammatory disorder characterized by noncardiogenic pulmonary edema, neutrophilic inflammation, and hypoxemia

### Noninfectious Causes of SIRS

Pancreatitis
Tissue trauma
Heat stroke
Ischemia
Burns
Pansystemic neoplasia

### Infectious Causes of SIRS (Sepsis)

Peritonitis
Pyometra
Prostatitis

Prostatic abscess
Pyelonephritis
Lower urinary tract infections
Pneumonia
Pyothorax
Gastroenteritis
Endocarditis
Nosocomial infections (IV catheters, urinary catheters, etc.)

## Clinical Findings of Sepsis and SIRS

Fever or hypothermia
Tachycardia, tachypnea
Neutrophilia with left shift or leukopenia
Anemia
Depression
Bounding or diminished pulses
Brick-red mucus membranes or pallor
Hypothermia
Thrombocytopenia
Hypoalbuminemia, hypoglycemia
DIC
Bilirubinemia
Elevated hepatic enzymes
Azotemia
Oliguria
Lactic acidosis
Hypoxemia
Signs related to underlying condition

## Vaccines, Recommended Core vs. Noncore

### Core Vaccines for Dogs

Distemper
Parvovirus
Adenovirus-2
Rabies

### Core Vaccines for Cats

Parvovirus (panleukopenia)
Herpesvirus-1
Calicivirus
Rabies

### Noncore Vaccines for Dogs

Need determined by individual clinician after assessment of
patient risk
• Bordetellosis

- Parainfluenza
- Canine influenza
- Leptospirosis
- Lyme borreliosis
- *Crotalus atrox*
- Canine influenza (strains H3N2 and H3N8)

### NONCORE VACCINES FOR CATS

Need determined by individual clinician after assessment of patient risk

- FeLV
- FIV
- *Chlamydophila felis* (formally, *Chlamydia psittaci*)
- Bordetellosis

## Viruses, Canine

## Common Viral Agents of Diseases of Dogs

### PARVOVIRUS

May be asymptomatic or fulminant disease

Anorexia, lethargy, fever, vomiting, hemorrhagic diarrhea, myocarditis (rare)

Worse in very young and parasitized puppies

Neutropenia, hypoalbuminemia, severe dehydration, secondary septicemia

### CORONAVIRUS

Diarrhea (infrequently blood in feces), vomiting, anorexia, lethargy, often self-limiting

Canine respiratory coronavirus, part of "kennel cough" complex

Coughing, sneezing, nasal discharge

Canine pancytotropic coronavirus

Severe clinical disease in puppies and juvenile dogs

Fever, lethargy, anorexia, vomiting, hemorrhagic diarrhea, ataxia, seizures

### ROTAVIRUS

Vomiting, diarrhea (rarely bloody), anorexia, typically recover after 5–7 days

### ADENOVIRUS TYPE 1 (INFECTIOUS CANINE HEPATITIS)

Fever, anorexia, lethargy, depression, abdominal pain, pale mucous membranes, tonsillitis, pharyngitis, coughing, hepatomegaly

Severe cases: coagulation abnormalities, petechiae, ecchymosis, DIC, rarely icterus, hepatic encephalopathy

Anterior uveitis and glomerulonephritis secondary to immune complex deposition

## CANINE DISTEMPER VIRUS

See Canine Distemper Virus Infection, Clinical Findings

## CANINE INFLUENZA A SUBTYPE H3N8 VIRUS, SUBTYPE H3N2

Acute onset of coughing, sneezing, nasal discharge, ocular discharge

Low-grade fever

Secondary commensal bacterial infections leading to mucopurulent discharge and productive cough

May lead to pneumonia with high fever, inappetence, productive cough, and increased respiratory effort

## RABIES VIRUS

Variable incubation period, prodromal phase: nervousness, anxiety, paresthesia

Progress to forebrain signs ("furious" form of rabies): irritability, restlessness, pica, photophobia, increased saliva production with decreasing ability to swallow, hyperesthesia progressing to incoordination, seizures, and death

May also progress to "dumb" form: paralysis, lower motor disease, leading to coma, respiratory paralysis, and death

## PSEUDORABIES

Suspected to be result from ingestion of infected raw pork

Neurologic dysfunction: ataxia, abnormal papillary light response, restlessness, trismus, cervical rigidity, ptyalism, tachypnea, excoriation from pruritus of head and neck; vomiting, diarrhea; most dogs die within 48 hours

## PARAINFLUENZA AND ADENOVIRUS TYPE 2

Hacking cough with gagging, easily elicited with tracheal palpation; cough may be paroxysmal, usually subsides within 7–10 days, and may lead to secondary bacterial or mycoplasmal infection

## CANINE HERPESVIRUS

Abortion, stillbirths; puppies born live progress to crying, hypothermia, soft stools, petechiae, cessation of nursing, and death

Older puppies develop mild respiratory signs that may emerge later as neurologic disease (ataxia, blindness, central vestibular disease)

Adult dogs: usually asymptomatic, rhinitis, pharyngitis, vaginal or preputial hyperemia, hyperplasia of vaginal mucosal lymphoid follicles, submucosal hemorrhage

## CANINE ORAL PAPILLOMAVIRUS
Oral papilloma (warts), may be quite extensive, spontaneously regress

## WEST NILE VIRUS
Clinical disease is uncommon.

## BORNAVIRUS
Seropositivity in the absence of clinical signs appears possible.

Tremors, salivation, mydriasis, circling

## Canine Distemper Virus Infection, Clinical Findings

### GENERAL SIGNS
Fever
Lethargy
Depression
Anorexia
Dehydration

### RESPIRATORY TRACT
Mucoid-to-mucopurulent discharge
Bronchopneumonia
- Coughing
- Crackles on auscultation
- Increased bronchovesicular sounds
- Dyspnea
Sneezing

### GASTROINTESTINAL TRACT
Vomiting
Small bowel diarrhea

### OCULAR DISEASE
Mucopurulent ocular discharge
Chorioretinitis, medallion lesions, optic neuritis, retinal detachment
Keratoconjunctivitis sicca
Anterior uveitis

### NEUROLOGIC DISEASE
Spinal cord lesion: paresis and ataxia
Central vestibular disease: head tilt, nystagmus, other CN and conscious proprioception deficits
Cerebellar disease: ataxia, head bobbing, hypermetria
Cerebral disease: seizures, blindness
Chorea myoclonus: rhythmic jerking of single muscles or muscle groups
Old dog encephalitis: ataxia, head pressing, pacing, hypermetric gait

### MISCELLANEOUS
Tonsillar enlargement
Pustular dermatosis
Hyperkeratosis of nose and footpads
Enamel hypoplasia

### IN UTERO INFECTION
Stillbirth
Abortion
"Fading puppy" syndrome in neonatal period
CNS signs at birth

## Viruses, Feline

### American Association of Feline Practitioners Guidelines for Retroviral Testing in Cats

Sick cats should be tested even if they have tested negative before.

Cats and kittens should be tested when they are first acquired.

Even cats not expected to live with other cats should be tested. This provides a health assessment of the individual; other cats may join the household; indoor cats may escape and expose other cats.

Tests should be performed at adoption, and negative cats should be retested a minimum of 60 days later.

Cats with known recent exposure to a retrovirus-infected cat or a cat with unknown status, particularly via a bite wound, should be tested regardless of previous test results. Testing should be done immediately and, if negative, should be repeated after a minimum of 60 days (when the type of potential viral exposure is unknown, retesting for both viruses after 60 days is most practical).

Cats living in households with other cats infected with FIV or FeLV should be tested annually.

High-risk cats (cats in cat-dense neighborhoods or cats that fight and get cat-bite wounds and abscesses) should be tested regularly.

Cats should be tested before initial vaccination against FeLV or FIV.

Always confirm an initial positive retrovirus test.

Cats used for blood or tissue donation should have negative screening tests for FeLV and FIV and should be negative for real-time PCR tests.

Intermittent retesting is not necessary for cats with confirmed negative infection status unless there is opportunity for exposure to infected cats or if they become ill.

Each cat should be individually tested. Testing of one cat as a proxy for another or pooling samples from multiple cats for testing is inappropriate.

## Clinical Signs of Rabies Virus Infection in Cats

Initially, signs are nonspecific: lethargy, inappetence, vomiting, diarrhea.

Rapid and continual deterioration of clinical conditions, no waxing and waning

Behavioral changes: more reclusive or attention seeking, may unpredictably attack animate, inanimate, or unseen objects

Irrevocable progression to classic signs, ptyalism with decreased ability to swallow leads to contamination of oral cavity, chin, and forelegs with potentially infectious saliva. CN signs such as anisocoria, pupil dysfunction, facial or tongue paresis, and changes in phonation may occur. Hyperesthesia and hyperresponsiveness to auditory and visual stimuli.

Auditory, visual, or tactile stimulation may elicit profound aggression to self-mutilation.

Become profoundly moribund to comatose to death; 100% fatal

## Feline Infectious Peritonitis (Feline Coronavirus Infection), Clinical Findings

### SIGNALMENT AND HISTORY

Purebred cats from cattery

Shelter environment

Multicat households

Younger than 5 years or older than 10 years of age

Previous history of mild, self-limiting GI or respiratory disease

Anorexia, weight loss, depression

Seizures, nystagmus, ataxia

Acute, fulminant course in cats with effusive FIP

Chronic, intermittent course in cats with noneffusive FIP; cats with the noneffusive form will commonly develop the effusive form later

The acute and chronic courses are different stages of the same disease, not separate forms, and both carry a poor prognosis.

### PHYSICAL EXAMINATION FINDINGS

Fever

Weight loss

Abdominal distension/fluid wave

Abdominal mass (focal intestinal granuloma, lymphadenopathy)

Icterus

Muffled heart or lung sounds

Dyspnea secondary to pleural effusion

Hepatomegaly

Chorioretinitis, iridocyclitis

Splenomegaly

Pale mucous membranes with or without petechiae

Multifocal neurologic abnormalities

Irregularly margined kidneys

Renomegaly

Ataxia, personality change, nystagmus, seizures

Rare presentations include skin fragility syndrome, orchitis, priaprism.

## CLINICOPATHOLOGIC ABNORMALITIES

CBC: nonregenerative anemia, neutrophilia with or without left shift, lymphopenia

Serum chemistry: elevated ALP and ALT, hyperbilirubinemia, hyperglobulinemia (polyclonal, rarely monoclonal gammopathy), azotemia (prerenal or renal)

Urinalysis: proteinuria

Nonseptic, pyogranulomatous exudate in peritoneal cavity, pleural space, and pericardium

Positive coronavirus antibody titer (especially in noneffusive cases)

CSF tap: increased protein concentration, neutrophilic pleocytosis, coronavirus antibodies

May see hydrocephalus with CT or magnetic resonance imaging (MRI) of the brain in cats with CNS FIP

Histopathology: pyogranulomatous inflammation in perivascular locations of tissues

Immunohistochemistry staining of FCoV antigen in macrophages of tissues (gold standard of diagnosis but requires tissue samples obtained by laparotomy, laparoscopy, or postmortem).

Positive for coronavirus on immunofluorescence or reverse transcriptase PCR (RT-PCR) testing of abdominal or pleural effusions (although these tests do not differentiate between FIP-causing viruses and "harmless" feline enteric coronavirus)

## FIV Infection, Clinical Findings

### PRIMARY PHASE OF INFECTION

Low-grade fever

Lymphadenopathy

Neutropenia

Often is unnoticed

Diagnosed often with screening tests in apparently
  healthy cats

**LATENT PHASE**
  No clinical signs for months to years

**IMMUNODEFICIENCY PHASE**
  Most cats never reach this phase.

  *Primary Viral Effects*
    Weight loss
    Nonregenerative anemia, neutropenia,
      thrombocytopenia
    Small bowel diarrhea
    Glomerulonephritis
    Myeloproliferative disorders
    Lymphoma
    Renal failure
    Anterior uveitis, pars planitis
    Behavioral abnormalities

  *Opportunistic Infectious Agents*
    Cutaneous: atypical mycobacteriosis, demodicosis,
      *Notoedres* and *Otodectes* infestation, dermato-
      phytosis, cryptococcosis, cowpox
    GI: cryptosporidiosis, coccidiosis, giardiasis, salmo-
      nellosis, campylobacteriosis, others
    Renal: bacterial infections, FIP, FeLV
    Urinary tract: bacterial infections
    Neoplasia: FeLV
    Hematologic: *Mycoplasma haemofelis*, FeLV,
      bartonellosis
    Neurologic: toxoplasmosis, cryptococcosis, FIP, FeLV
    Ophthalmologic: toxoplasmosis, FIP, cryptococcosis,
      herpesvirus, bartonellosis
    Pneumonia/pneumonitis: bacterial, toxoplasmosis,
      cryptococcosis
    Pyothorax: bacterial
    Stomatitis: calicivirus, bacterial, candidiasis,
      bartonellosis
    Upper respiratory: herpesvirus, calicivirus, bacterial,
      cryptococcosis

## FeLV, Clinical Findings

**ACUTE PHASE**
  Fever
  Malaise
  Diarrhea
  Leukopenia

## GENERAL SIGNS
Anorexia
Weight loss
Depression
Many FeLV-positive cats are asymptomatic at diagnosis, found incidentally with routine screening.

## NEOPLASTIC
Lymphoma: mediastinal, multicentric, alimentary, renal
Leukemia: lymphocytic, myelogenous, erythroid, megakaryocytic
Myeloproliferative disorders
Fibrosarcoma

## ICTERUS
Prehepatic: immune-mediated RBC destruction induced by FeLV or secondary infection with *Mycoplasma haemofelis*
Hepatic: hepatic lymphoma, focal liver necrosis, hepatic lipidosis
Posthepatic: alimentary lymphoma

## BONE MARROW
Pure red cell aplasia
Regenerative anemia (less common and often associated with coinfection with *Mycoplasma haemofelis*)
Myeloproliferative disease (anemia, leukopenia, thrombocytopenia)

## STOMATITIS
Bacterial infection
Calicivirus infection

## RHINITIS/PNEUMONIA
Bacteria
Herpesvirus and calicivirus

## RENAL
Glomerulonephritis
Renal failure
Urinary incontinence: sphincter incompetence or detrusor hyperactivity

## OCULAR LYMPHOMA
Aqueous flare, mass lesions, keratitic precipitates, lens luxations, glaucoma, anterior uveitis

## NEUROLOGIC POLYNEUROPATHY OR LYMPHOMA
Anisocoria, ataxia, weakness, tetraparesis, paraparesis, behavioral changes, urinary incontinence
Secondary infection with FIP, *Toxoplasma gondii*, *Cryptococcus neoformans*

## IN UTERO INFECTION

Abortion, stillbirth, infertility, kitten mortality complex ("fading kitten" syndrome)

## LAMENESS

Neutrophilic polyarthritis secondary to immune complex deposition

Multiple cartilaginous exostoses

## FeLV, Possible Outcomes After Exposure

### PROGRESSIVE INFECTION

Viral replication in lymphoid tissue and bone marrow, spread to mucosal and glandular tissues, leading to shedding of virus. Most cats become persistently infected and frequently die of an FeLV-associated disease within a few years. Antigen (ELISA) and provirus (PCR) positive.

### REGRESSIVE INFECTION

Effective immune response limits viral replication. FeLV antigen detectable in peripheral blood within 2–3 weeks after exposure but disappears 2–8 weeks later. Provirus positive on PCR, antibody positive. May not ever develop antigenemia. Clinical relevance of regressive infection is not clear. May have persistent integration of FeLV DNA in their genome but are unlikely to develop FeLV-associated diseases. Do not shed virus.

### ABORTIVE EXPOSURE

Characterized by negative results for culturable virus, antigen, viral RNA, and proviral DNA (PCR). These cats are healthy and not contagious, and likely have lifelong protection from new infection.

### FOCAL INFECTIONS

Rare events in which cats have FeLV infection restricted to certain tissues such as spleen, lymph nodes, small intestine, or mammary glands

## Other Feline Viral Diseases

### UPPER RESPIRATORY TRACT VIRUSES

Herpesvirus type 1: ocular and nasal disease

Calicivirus: ocular, nasal, and oral disease; rarely, joint disease

Reovirus: conjunctivitis, respiratory lesions, diarrhea experimentally, no evidence of importance in the field

### ENTERIC VIRUSES

Feline parvovirus (panleukopenia virus): enteritis, panleukopenia, cerebellar hypoplasia, fetal death

Feline coronavirus: mild enteritis, FIP

Rotavirus: rare cause of mild diarrhea

Astrovirus: uncommon cause of persistent watery diarrhea

Torovirus: may be associated with protruding nictitating membrane and diarrhea syndrome

## MISCELLANEOUS

Cowpox virus: mainly see skin lesions; sporadic disease in cats

Hantavirus: zoonotic disease of wild rodents; clinical significance in cats not known

Rabies virus

Pseudorabies virus: cats are a rare host, severe behavioral changes, pruritus, paralysis, coma, death

Feline herpesvirus type 2: possible association with feline idiopathic lower urinary tract disease

# Joint and Bone Disorders

Arthritis
Bone Disorders

## Arthritis

### Differential Diagnosis: Infectious Arthritis

#### SEPTIC ARTHRITIS
*Bacterial Suppurative Arthritis*
Penetrating wounds
- Animal bites

Iatrogenic
- Infection during surgery, arthrocentesis

Trauma (e.g., hit by car)
Hematogenous
- Endocarditis
- Omphalophlebitis
- Pyoderma
- Other foci of infection

#### LYME ARTHRITIS
*Borrelia burgdorferi*
Transmitted by *Ixodes* ticks
Illness in cats is rare

#### BACTERIAL L-FORM ARTHRITIS
Cell wall–deficient bacteria
Causes suppurative arthritis and subcutaneous abscesses
  in cats

#### *MYCOPLASMA* ARTHRITIS
Debilitated and immunosuppressed animals
*M. gatae, M. felis* in cats

#### FUNGAL ARTHRITIS (RARE)
*Coccidioides immitis*
*Blastomyces dermatitidis*
*Cryptococcus neoformans*
*Sporothrix schenckii*
*Aspergillus terreus*

#### RICKETTSIAL ARTHRITIS
Rocky Mountain spotted fever *(Rickettsia rickettsii)*
*Ehrlichia canis*
*Anaplasma phagocytophilum*

### PROTOZOAL ARTHRITIS
Leishmaniasis (*Leishmania* spp.)
Toxoplasmosis (rare)
Neosporosis *(Neospora caninum):* polyarthritis, poly-
myositis, neurologic disease
Hepatozoonosis: polyarthritis and polymyositis in dog
and cat
Babesiosis (rare, more often causes severe anemia)
Chlamydiae (feline)

### VIRAL ARTHRITIS
Calicivirus infection in cats

## Differential Diagnosis of Noninfectious Arthritis

### NONEROSIVE
Immune-mediated polyarthritis; most cases are
idiopathic
SLE
Reactive polyarthritis (bacterial, fungal, para-
sitic, neoplastic, enterohepatic, drug reaction,
vaccine–induced)
Breed-associated syndromes
Polyarthritis (Akita, Newfoundland, Weimaraner)
Polyarthritis/meningitis (Akita, Beagle, Bernese
Mountain Dog, Boxer, German Shorthaired Pointer)
Polyarthritis/polymyositis (spaniels)
Familial Shar-Pei fever
Lymphoplasmacytic synovitis
Osteoarthritis (secondary to trauma, joint instability,
incongruity, immobilization, or osteochondrosis)

### EROSIVE
Rheumatoid-like arthritis
Erosive polyarthritis of Greyhounds
Feline chronic progressive polyarthritis

## Bone Disorders

## Differential Diagnosis: Congenital, Developmental, Genetic

### CONGENITAL
Hemimelia, phocomelia, amelia: absence of portions or
entire limb (amelia)
Syndactyly: fusion of two or more digits; rarely clinically
significant
Polydactyly: extra digits

Ectrodactyly: third metacarpal and digit missing,
    forming a cleft (split or "lobster claw")
Segmented hemiatrophy: limb hypoplasia

## DEVELOPMENTAL AND GENETIC

Osteopetrosis: rare; diaphysis remains filled with bone,
    marrow does not form, fragile bones
Osteogenesis imperfecta: heritable diseases—fragile bones
Mucopolysaccharidosis: rare lysosomal storage disease—
    Siamese cats—causes dwarfism, facial dysmorphism
Dwarfism
- Osteochondrodysplasias
- Pituitary dwarfism
- Congenital hypothyroidism
Retained cartilage cores
Craniomandibular osteopathy (West Highland White
    Terrier, Scottish Terrier, Cairn Terrier, Boston Terrier,
    other terriers)
Multiple cartilaginous exostoses
Avascular necrosis of the femoral head

# Differential Diagnosis: Metabolic, Nutritional, Endocrine, Idiopathic

## METABOLIC

Nutritional secondary hyperparathyroidism
Lead poisoning

## NUTRITIONAL

Rickets (hypovitaminosis D)
Renal osteodystrophy
Hypervitaminosis A: causes osteopathy
Hypovitaminosis A: deformed bones secondary to
    impedance of bone remodeling
Hypervitaminosis D: skeletal demineralization
Zinc-responsive chondrodysplasia
Copper deficiency
Overnutrition of growing dogs

## ENDOCRINE

Primary hyperparathyroidism
Humoral hypercalcemia of malignancy
Hyperadrenocorticism
Hypogonadism: delay in physis closure after early
    gonadectomy
Hepatic osteodystrophy
Anticonvulsant osteodystrophy

## IDIOPATHIC

Enostosis (panosteitis)
Metaphyseal osteopathy (hypertrophic osteodystrophy)
Avascular necrosis of femoral head (Legg-Calvé-Perthes disease)
Secondary hypertrophic osteopathy (usually in response to thoracic neoplasia)
Medullary bone infarction
Bone cyst
Aneurysmal bone cyst
Subchondral bone cyst
Fibrous dysplasia
Central giant cell granuloma
Carpal laxity syndrome (giant-breed 6–12 week-old puppies)

# Liver and Exocrine Pancreatic Disorders

## Cholangitis and Cholangiohepatitis, Feline

### Comparative Clinical Findings

#### SUPPURATIVE (NEUTROPHILIC) CHOLANGITIS AND CHOLANGIOHEPATITIS

Middle-aged to older cats

Often depressed and ill

Anorexia (usually)

Vomiting

Abdominal discomfort

Jaundice

Neutrophilia

Increased ALT

Increased ALP

Increased bilirubin (±)

Increased serum and urine bile acids (±)

Abnormal coagulation values

Hyperechoic liver, gallbladder distension, cholelithiasis, biliary sludge, thickened gallbladder wall, cystic and common bile duct dilation and tortuosity, ascites

Primarily neutrophilic infiltrate

Lesions surround bile ducts

May be associated with pancreatitis and/or inflammatory bowel disease (triaditis)

Respond to antibiotics and supportive nonspecific treatments

223

## LYMPHOCYTIC CHOLANGITIS

Younger cats

Persians

Bright and alert

Polyphagia (±)

Ascites (±)

Icterus (±)

Fever (±)

Lymphadenopathy (±)

Hepatomegaly (±)

Neutrophilia (±)

Lymphopenia (±)

Bile acids (±)

Increased ALT

Increased ALP

Bilirubinemia/bilirubinuria (±)

Hyperglobulinemia (most consistent biochemical abnormality)

Hyperechoic liver, gallbladder distension, cholelithiasis, biliary sludge, thickened gallbladder wall, cystic and common bile duct dilation and tortuosity, ascites (±)

Primarily lymphocytic infiltrate

Lesions found in portal areas

Variable fibrosis

Pancreatitis (may be present)

Positive response to immunosuppressive corticosteroids

## Exocrine Pancreatic Disease

### Differential Diagnosis

Pancreatitis
- Acute
- Chronic

EPI

Pancreatic pseudocyst

Pancreatic abscess

Exocrine pancreatic neoplasia
- Pancreatic adenoma
- Pancreatic adenocarcinoma
- Pancreatic sarcoma (spindle cell sarcoma, lymphosarcoma) rare

Nodular hyperplasia

Pancreatic parasites (cats)
- *Eurytrema procyonis* (pancreatic fluke)
- *Amphimerus pseudofelineus* (hepatic fluke)

Pancreatic bladder
- Abnormal extension of pancreatic duct (rare finding in cat)

## Clinical Findings of Exocrine Pancreatic Insufficiency

Most often seen in young to middle-aged dogs; German Shepherds are predisposed; less common but is seen in cats

Chronic weight loss

Ravenous appetite (cats with EPI can present with decreased appetite)

Coprophagia

Pica

Change in fecal character
- Voluminous
- Soft
- Watery
- Color change
- May be normal

Poor hair coat quality

Borborygmus, flatulence

Coagulation disorder (caused by malabsorption of vitamin K, rare)

## Gallbladder and Extrahepatic Biliary Disease

### Differential Diagnosis

#### OBSTRUCTIVE DISEASE

Extrahepatic biliary obstruction
- Pancreatitis (most common etiology in dog)
- Biliary neoplasia
- Cholangitis
- Pancreatic neoplasia

Cholelithiasis/choledocholithiasis

Gallbladder mucocele

#### NONOBSTRUCTIVE DISEASE

Cholecystitis
- Bacterial cholecystitis (ascending infection—*Escherichia coli* most common)
- Necrotizing cholecystitis
- Emphysematous cholecystitis (*E. coli, Clostridium perfringens*)

Cholelithiasis/choledocholithiasis (does not always cause obstruction)

Parasites (mainly seen in cats)

Tropical climates (seen in cats that eat lizards or toads)
- *Platynosomum fastosum* (a fluke)
- *Amphimerus pseudofelineus*
- *Metorchis conjunctus*
- *Eurytrema procyonis*

Gallbladder infarct

## NEOPLASIA
Biliary cystadenoma
Bile duct carcinoma

## CAROLI DISEASE
Congenital dilatation of intra- and extrahepatic bile ducts and diffuse cystic kidney disease reported in dogs

## GALLBLADDER RUPTURE
Necrotizing cholecystitis
Obstruction
Iatrogenic
Blunt abdominal trauma
Gallbladder torsion
Dogs with hypothyroidism and hyperadrenocorticism may be predisposed to infarct/rupture

# Clinical Findings of Gallbladder and Biliary Disease

## CLINICAL SIGNS
Vomiting
Icterus
Anorexia
Fever
Abdominal pain
Depression
Weight loss
Ascites/bile peritonitis

## CLINICOPATHOLOGIC FINDINGS
Hyperbilirubinemia
Elevated ALP levels
Elevated gamma glutamyltransferase (GGT) levels
Elevated serum bile acids
Elevated ALT levels
Hypercholesterolemia
Stress leukogram
Nonregenerative anemia

## RADIOGRAPHIC FINDINGS
Hepatomegaly
Mass effect in area of gallbladder
Gas shadow in area of gallbladder

Choleliths radiopaque if they contain calcium (50% may not be seen on radiographs)

## ULTRASONOGRAPHIC SIGNS

Dilated and tortuous bile ducts

Gallbladder distension

Thickened gallbladder wall

Cholelith visible

Free abdominal fluid with gallbladder rupture

Pancreatic mass identified

Stellate appearance to contents of gallbladder (characteristic of a gallbladder mucocele)

## Hepatic Encephalopathy

## Clinical Findings

### GENERAL SYSTEMIC CLINICAL SIGNS

Anorexia

Depression

Weight loss

Lethargy

Nausea

Fever

Ptyalism

Intermittent vomiting

Diarrhea

Polyuria/polydipsia

Stranguria, pollakiuria, hematuria (biurate urolithiasis)

### CENTRAL NERVOUS SYSTEM CLINICAL SIGNS

Tremors

Ataxia

Personality change (often toward aggression)

Dementia

Head pressing

Pacing

Circling

Cortical blindness

Seizures

Coma

## Hepatic Lipidosis, Feline

## Clinical Findings

### HISTORICAL FINDINGS

Obesity

Recent anorexia and rapid weight loss

- Concurrent disease that causes anorexia (pancreatitis, diabetes mellitus, inflammatory hepatobiliary disease, inflammatory bowel disease, FIP, chronic renal failure, neoplasia, cardiomyopathy, neurologic disease, etc.)
- Stressful event
- Abrupt diet change

Typically indoor cats

## PHYSICAL FINDINGS

Jaundice
Vomiting
Dehydration
Hepatic encephalopathy
- Depression
- Ptyalism

Hepatomegaly

## CLINICOPATHOLOGIC FINDINGS

Typical findings of cholestasis
- Moderate increase in ALT
- Marked increase in ALP
- Mild increase in GGT; disproportionately low compared with other feline cholestatic hepatopathies
- Elevated serum bile acids typical, not useful in icteric patients
- Bilirubinuria

Coagulation test abnormalities (especially in conjunction with acute pancreatitis)

Abdominal ultrasound = normal-to-increased liver size, diffusely hyperechoic parenchyma

## CYTOLOGY (ULTRASOUND-GUIDED NEEDLE ASPIRATES) AND HISTOPATHOLOGY

Reveal clear vacuolation of most hepatocytes, nonzonal in distribution; typically with absence of inflammatory cells

## Hepatobiliary Disease

## Clinical and Physical Findings

### GENERAL CLINICAL FEATURES

Depression
Anorexia
Lethargy
Weight loss
Poor hair coat, insufficient grooming
Nausea, vomiting

Diarrhea
Dehydration
Small body stature
Polydipsia, polyuria

## SIGNS SPECIFIC BUT NOT PATHOGNOMONIC FOR HEPATIC DISEASE

Icterus
Bilirubinuria
Acholic feces
Organomegaly
Ascites
Hepatic encephalopathy
- Behavioral changes (aggression, dementia, hysteria)
- Circling
- Ataxia
- Staggering
- Pacing
- Head pressing
- Cortical blindness
- Ptyalism
- Tremors/seizures
- Coma
Coagulopathies
Polydipsia/polyuria

## Causes of Elevated Serum Hepatobiliary Enzymes

### PRIMARY HEPATIC DISEASE

### DRUG INDUCTION

Corticosteroids (dogs)
Anticonvulsants (phenobarbital, phenytoin, primidone)

### ENDOCRINOPATHIES

Hyperadrenocorticism (dogs)
Hypothyroidism (dogs)
Hyperthyroidism (cats)
Diabetes mellitus

### BONE DISORDERS

Growing animals
Osteosarcoma
Osteomyelitis

### NEOPLASIA

Adenocarcinomas (pancreatic, intestinal, adrenocortical, mammary)
Sarcomas (hemangiosarcoma, leiomyosarcoma)
Hepatic metastasis

### MUSCLE INJURY
Acute muscle necrosis/trauma
Myopathies
Malignant hyperthermia

### HYPOXIA/HYPOTENSION
Septic shock
Surgery
CHF
Hypoadrenocorticism
Circulatory shock
Severe acute blood loss
Hypotensive crisis
Status epilepticus

### GASTROINTESTINAL DISEASE
Pancreatitis
Inflammatory bowel disease

### MISCELLANEOUS CAUSES
Systemic infections
Pregnancy (cats—increased placental ALP)
Colostrum-fed neonates (dogs)
Breed-related (Scottish Terrier)

## Differential Diagnosis, Dogs

### INFLAMMATION
Chronic hepatitis complex
- Copper accumulation—Bedlington Terrier, Airedale Terrier, Bull Terrier, Bulldog, Cocker Spaniel, Collie, Dachshund, Dalmatian, Doberman Pinscher, German Shepherd, Golden Retriever, Keeshond, Kerry Blue Terrier, Labrador Retriever, Norwich Terrier, Old English Sheepdog, Pekingese, Poodle, Samoyed, Schnauzer, Skye Terrier, West Highland White Terrier, Wire Fox Terrier
- Drug-induced: trimethoprim-sulfa, phenobarbital, diethylcarbamazine, oxibendazole, many others
- Familial hepatitis—Doberman Pinscher, West Highland White Terrier, Dalmatian, Skye Terrier, Cocker Spaniel

Fibrosis and cirrhosis (results from any severe or chronic hepatic insult)

Infectious agents: leptospirosis, canine adenovirus type 1 infection, bacterial hepatitis, histoplasmosis, Rocky Mountain spotted fever, ehrlichiosis, babesiosis, leishmaniasis

Cholangiohepatitis
Granulomatous hepatitis
- *Rhodococcus, Borrelia, Bartonella, Histoplasma, Coccidioidomyces, Hepatozoon, Heterobilharzia, Nocardia, Mycobacterium* spp.

Acidophil cell hepatitis
Lobular dissecting hepatitis
Hepatic abscess

## ACUTE TOXIC OR DRUG-INDUCED HEPATOPATHY

## VACUOLAR HEPATOPATHY

## METABOLIC LIVER DISEASE
Amyloidosis
Hyperlipidemia
Lysosomal storage disease

## VASCULAR HEPATIC DISEASE
Congenital portosystemic venous anomaly
Intrahepatic portal vein hypoplasia
Intrahepatic arteriovenous fistula

## BILIARY TRACT DISEASE

## NEOPLASIA
Primary: hepatocellular carcinoma, hepatocellular adenoma, hepatic hemangiosarcoma, biliary carcinoma
Other hepatic tumors: leiomyosarcoma, liposarcoma, myxosarcoma, fibrosarcoma, biliary adenoma, hepatic carcinoid
Hemolymphatic: lymphosarcoma, MCT, plasma cell tumor
Metastatic neoplasia

## HEPATIC OR BILIARY CYSTS

## Differential Diagnosis, Cats

### HEPATIC LIPIDOSIS

### INFLAMMATORY HEPATOBILIARY DISEASE
Cholangitis/cholangiohepatitis complex
- Suppurative (neutrophilic) cholangitis, cholangiohepatitis
- Lymphocytic cholangitis

Chronic cholangiohepatitis (later stage of acute cholangiohepatitis)
Sclerosing cholangitis
Lymphocytic portal hepatitis
FIP

## TOXIC HEPATOPATHY
Antimicrobials (trimethoprim-sulfa, tetracycline)
Anticonvulsants (phenobarbital)
Diazepam
Methimazole
Griseofulvin
Ketoconazole
Pine oils (cleaning agents)
NSAIDs
*Amanita phalloides* (death cap mushroom)
Natural or herbal remedies
Many others

## PORTOSYSTEMIC VENOUS ANOMALY

## LIPOPROTEIN LIPASE DEFICIENCY

## NEOPLASIA
*Primary Hepatic Neoplasia*
Biliary carcinoma
Hepatocellular carcinoma
Hepatic hemangiosarcoma
Biliary cystadenoma
Myelolipoma
Hepatic carcinoid

*Hemolymphatic Neoplasia*
Lymphosarcoma
MCT
Plasma cell tumor

*Metastatic Neoplasia*

## Hepatomegaly and Microhepatica

## Differential Diagnosis

### GENERALIZED HEPATOMEGALY
Acute toxic hepatopathy
Infiltrative hepatic disease
- Neoplasia: primary or metastatic
- Chronic hepatitis complex (dog)
- Cholangitis/cholangiohepatitis (cat)
- Extramedullary hematopoiesis
- Mononuclear-phagocytic cell hyperplasia
- Amyloidosis (rare)
- Hepatic lipidosis (cat)
Passive congestion
- Right-sided heart failure
- Pericardial disease (dog)

- Caval syndrome (dog)
- Caudal vena cava obstruction (dog)
- Budd-Chiari syndrome (rare)

Hepatocellular hypertrophy

- Hepatic lipidosis
- Steroid hepatopathy
- Hyperadrenocorticism
- Anticonvulsant drug therapy

Acute extrahepatic bile duct obstruction

### FOCAL HEPATOMEGALY

Neoplasia: primary or metastatic

Nodular hyperplasia

Chronic hepatic disease with fibrosis and nodular regeneration

Hepatic abscess

Hepatic cyst

### MICROHEPATICA

Decreased hepatic mass

- Chronic hepatic disease with progressive loss of hepatocytes

Decreased portal blood flow with hepatocellular atrophy

- Congenital portosystemic shunt
- Intrahepatic portal vein hypoplasia
- Chronic portal vein thrombosis
- Hepatic microvascular dysplasia

Hypovolemia

- Hypoadrenocorticism
- Shock

## Hyperlipidemia

### Differential Diagnosis

#### POSTPRANDIAL HYPERLIPIDEMIA

*Primary*

Idiopathic hyperlipoproteinemia of Miniature Schnauzers

Feline familial hyperchylomicronemia

Idiopathic hypercholesterolemia (rare—Doberman Pinscher, Rottweiler)

*Secondary*

Endocrine

- Hypothyroidism
- Diabetes mellitus
- Hyperadrenocorticism

Pancreatitis
Protein-losing nephropathy
Hepatic insufficiency
Cholestasis
Drug-induced
- Glucocorticoids
- Megestrol acetate
- Phenobarbital

## Clinical Findings

### SEVERE HYPERLIPIDEMIA

Intermittent GI signs
- Vomiting
- Diarrhea
- Abdominal discomfort

Seizures
Pancreatitis
Lipemia retinalis
Uveitis
Cutaneous xanthomas
Peripheral nerve paralysis
Behavioral changes

### SEVERE HYPERCHOLESTEROLEMIA

Arcus lipoides corneae
Lipemia retinalis
Atherosclerosis

## Pancreatitis

## Clinical Findings of Acute Pancreatitis

### DOGS

#### *Mild Acute Pancreatitis*

Depression
Anorexia
Nausea, vomiting, diarrhea
Ptyalism
Mild right cranial-abdominal pain
Fever, dehydration, weakness

#### *Moderate-to-Severe Acute Pancreatitis*

Depression
Anorexia
Vomiting
Right cranial abdominal pain
Hematemesis, hematochezia, melena
Jaundice

Respiratory distress
Shock, fever, dehydration
Hyperemic mucous membranes
Tachycardia, tachypnea
Abdominal effusion
Mass effect in region of pancreas
Petechiae, ecchymoses
Cardiac arrhythmia
Glossitis, glossal slough
Extrahepatic biliary obstruction

### CATS

Signs tend to be more subclinical and nonspecific.
May be associated with inflammatory bowel disease
May be component of multisystemic disease such as
toxoplasmosis
Lethargy, anorexia, vomiting, dehydration, weight loss,
jaundice, hypothermia
Rarely icterus, abdominal pain
May present as acute necrotizing or acute suppurative
form

## Predisposing Factors

### NUTRITIONAL

Obesity
High-fat diet
After ingestion of large, fatty meal or dietary
indiscretion

### HYPERTRIGLYCERIDEMIA

### HYPERLIPOPROTEINEMIA (IDIOPATHIC IN MINIATURE SCHNAUZERS)

Endocrine (diabetes mellitus, hyperadrenocorticism,
hypothyroidism)

### DRUGS

Chemotherapeutic agents
- L-asparaginase
- Azathioprine
- Others
Organophosphates
Asparaginase
Thiazides
Furosemide
Estrogens
Sulfa drugs
Phenobarbital
Procainamide

Potassium bromide
Tetracyclines
Corticosteroids do not seem to be implicated.

### ISCHEMIA
Hypovolemia
Associated with DIC
Vasoactive amine–induced vasoconstriction
Surgery
Gastric dilatation/volvulus
Severe immune-mediated hemolytic anemia

### DUODENAL REFLUX
Increased intraluminal pressure during severe vomiting

### OTHER
Cholangitis
Infection (toxoplasmosis, FIP)
Abdominal trauma
Hypercalcemia
Trauma

## Clinicopathologic Findings in Dogs and Cats With Acute Pancreatitis

BUN/creatinine—increased in 50%–65% of dogs and in
33% (Cr) and 57% (BUN) in cats. Usually prerenal due
to dehydration and hypotension. May be secondary to
intrinsic renal failure (sepsis and immune complex).

Potassium—decreased in 20% of cases in dogs and 56% in
cats. Increased loss in vomiting and due to renal loss with
fluid therapy plus reduced intake and aldosterone release
caused by hypovolemia.

Sodium—can be increased, decreased, or normal. Increase
usually caused by dehydration, decrease caused by losses
secondary to vomiting.

Calcium—commonly decreased in cats, rarely in dogs,
rarely increased in both dogs and cats. Reduction is a poor
prognostic indicator in cats but has no prognostic significance in dogs. May be caused by saponification in peri-
pancreatic fat and glucagon release stimulating calcitonin.

Chloride—very commonly decreased in dogs. Loss in GI
secretions in vomiting.

Phosphate—often increased in dogs; uncommonly
increased or decreased in cats. Increase usually due to
reduced renal excretion secondary to renal compromise.
Decrease (in cats) due to treatment for diabetes mellitus.

Glucose—increased in 40%–88% of dogs and decreased in up
to 40%. Increased in 64% of cats, rarely decreased. Increase

due to decreased insulin and increased glucagon, cortisol, and catecholamines. Decrease caused by sepsis or anorexia.

Albumin—increased in 39%–50% and decreased in 17% of dogs. Increased in 8%–30% and decreased in 40% of cats. Increase due to dehydration. Decrease due to gut loss, malnutrition, concurrent hepatic disease, or renal loss.

Hepatocellular enzymes (ALT, AST)—increased in 61% of dogs and 68% of cats. Hepatic necrosis and vacuolation due to sepsis, local effects of pancreatitis, ± concurrent hepatic disease in cats.

Cholestatic enzymes (ALP and GGT)—increased in 79% of dogs and 50% of cats. Biliary obstruction due to acute or chronic pancreatitis ± concurrent cholangitis ± lipidosis in cats; steroid-induced ALP in dogs.

Bilirubin—increased in 53% of dogs and 64% of cats (same causes as GGT and ALP).

Cholesterol—increased in 48%–80% of dogs and 64% of cats. Can be due to cholestasis; unclear if cause or effect.

Triglycerides—commonly increased in dogs. Unclear if cause or effect.

Neutrophils—increased in 55%–60% of dogs, increased in 30% and decreased in 15% of cats. Increased due to inflammatory response. Decreased in some cats due to consumption; may be a poor prognostic indicator.

Hematocrit—increased in about 20% and decreased in 20% of both dogs and cats. Increased due to dehydration and decreased due to anemia of chronic disease or gastric ulceration.

Platelets—commonly decreased in severe cases in dogs. Decreased due to circulating proteases ± DIC.

## Portosystemic Shunt, Congenital and Acquired

### Congenital—May be Intrahepatic (More Common in Large-Breed Dogs) or Extrahepatic (More Common in Small Dogs and Cats)

#### ACQUIRED—NO BREED OR GENDER PREDILECTION

*Clinical Findings*

Signalment

Young animal, male or female, often purebred

History

Neurologic signs (dementia, circling, central blindness, personality change, head pressing, wall hugging, seizures)

Vomiting

Diarrhea

Ptyalism (especially cats)
Worsening of signs after eating
Improvement of signs with antimicrobial therapy
Prolonged recovery from anesthesia
Polydipsia/polyuria
Recurrent urate urolithiasis in breeds other than Dalmatian and English Bulldog

Physical Examination
Poor hair coat
Small stature
Cystic calculi
Cryptorchidism
Bilateral renomegaly
Copper-colored irises in non-Asian cat breeds
Other congenital anomalies

## CLINICOPATHOLOGIC FINDINGS

Microcytosis
Hypoalbuminemia
Mild increases in hepatic enzymes
Hypocholesterolemia
Low BUN
Normal-to-high resting bile acids/elevated postprandial bile acids
Hyposthenuria
Urate crystalluria and urolithiasis

## Vacuolar Hepatopathy, Canine

### Differential Diagnosis

Hyperadrenocorticism
- Pituitary-dependent
- Adrenal-dependent
- Iatrogenic (glucocorticoid therapy)

Pancreatitis
- Chronic

Severe hypothyroidism

Chronic stress
- Illness of more than 4 months

Chronic infection or inflammation (e.g., pyelonephritis, chronic dermatitis)

Severe dental disease
- Oral infection

Disorders affecting lipid metabolism
- Diabetes mellitus
- Idiopathic hyperlipidemia

Neoplasia
- Lymphoma

CHF

Toxicosis (e.g., aflatoxin)

Abnormal sex hormone production

Inflammatory bowel disease
- Chronic, lymphoplasmacytic, eosinophilic

Hepatocutaneous syndrome

# Neoplasia

## Chemotherapeutic Agent Toxicity

Most severely affects tissues with a growth fraction that approaches that of tumor cells

### Clinical Findings

**MYELOSUPPRESSION**

Neutropenia: short-lived cells; nadir is 5–10 days postchemotherapy

Thrombocytopenia: nadir is 7–14 days postchemotherapy

Anemia: erythrocytes live longer; rarely clinically significant

**GASTROINTESTINAL TOXICITY**

Nausea, vomiting

Diarrhea

Inappetence

Anorexia

**CARDIOTOXICITY**

Doxorubicin therapy

Breeds susceptible to dilated cardiomyopathy (e.g., Doberman Pinscher) most sensitive

Most likely after cumulative dose of $180\,mg/m^2$

**NEPHROTOXICITY**

Cisplatin, streptozotocin, toceranib

Limit use of cisplatin in cases of preexisting renal disease

**HEPATOPATHY**

Irreversible hepatic toxicity may result if lomustine (CCNU) given in face of elevated ALT

## UROTHELIAL TOXICITY
Sterile hemorrhagic cystitis
Cyclophosphamide, ifosfamide

## EXTRAVASATION
Doxorubicin: severe local reaction leading to slough
Vincristine: usually minor tissue damage

## HYPERSENSITIVITY
Doxorubicin: caused by histamine release from mast cells; prevented by slow administration
L-asparaginase: less likely if given subcutaneously rather than intravenously
Etoposide, paclitaxel: caused by carrier solutions for these agents

## ALOPECIA
Less of a problem in dogs and cats than in people
Worse in breeds that have hair (e.g., Poodles, Terriers, Old English Sheepdogs) than in dogs with fur
Loss of "feathers" (e.g., Golden Retrievers)
Loss of whiskers in cats

## PANCREATITIS

## NEUROLOGIC TOXICITY
Fatal neurotoxicity in cats with topical or systemic administration of 5-fluorouracil

## RESPIRATORY TOXICITY
Fatal, acute pulmonary edema in cats with cisplatin therapy

## Corticosteroid Therapy

## Adverse Effects Associated With Glucocorticoid Administration

Polyuria/polydipsia
Polyphagia
Increased ALP levels
Increased GGT levels
Panting
Insomnia, agitation, behavioral changes
Immunosuppression
- Secondary infection
- Recrudescence of latent infection
- Worsening of existing infection
- Demodicosis

Vacuolar hepatopathy
Iatrogenic hyperadrenocorticism
Adrenocorticoid deficiency with rapid withdrawal after
  sustained use
Alopecia
Calcinosis cutis
Comedones
Skin thinning
Proteinuria
Muscle atrophy/muscle wasting
Myotonia/myopathy
Delayed wound healing
Colonic perforation
GI ulceration
Insulin resistance
Diabetes mellitus
Hyperlipidemia
Abortion
Growth suppression
Hypercoagulable state
Ligament and tendon rupture
Psychosis/behavior change
Lowered seizure threshold
Osteopenia

## Histiocytic Disease

### Classification, Dogs

May be difficult to differentiate from lymphoproliferative,
  granulomatous, or reactive inflammatory disease by histopathology alone

#### CUTANEOUS HISTIOCYTOMA

Benign, usually solitary lesion
Typically young dogs
Often spontaneously regress

#### LANGERHANS CELL HISTIOCYTOMA

Rare, rapidly metastatic, cutaneous infiltration by his-
  tiocytes, may be limited to multiple cutaneous sites or
  may affect lymph nodes and internal organs

#### CUTANEOUS HISTIOCYTOSIS

Single or multiple lesions
May spontaneously regress
May respond to immunosuppressive drugs

## SYSTEMIC HISTIOCYTOSIS

Familial disease of Bernese Mountain Dogs, rarely other breeds

Similar lesions to cutaneous histiocytosis, but may also affect mucous membranes, lymphoid organs, lung, bone marrow, and other organ systems

Progressive, requires immunosuppressive therapy

## HISTIOCYTIC SARCOMA

Bernese Mountain Dog, Rottweiler, Flat-Coated Retriever, Golden Retriever, rarely other breeds

Histiocytic sarcoma usually begins as a localized lesion in spleen, lymph nodes, lung, bone marrow, skin and subcutis, brain, and periarticular tissue of appendicular joints

- Rapidly disseminates to multiple organs

## MALIGNANT HISTIOCYTOSIS

Bernese Mountain Dog, Rottweiler, Flat-Coated Retriever, Golden Retriever, rarely other breeds

Multisystemic, rapidly progressive disease of multiple organs

## Classification, Cats

### FELINE PROGRESSIVE HISTIOCYTOSIS

Rare, usually see multiple skin nodules, papules, plaques

Head, lower extremities, trunk

Poor long-term prognosis

### FELINE HISTIOCYTIC SARCOMA

Poorly demarcated tumors of subcutis or spleen

Poor prognosis

## Humoral Hypercalcemia

## Differential Diagnosis

### HEMATOLOGIC CANCERS

Lymphosarcoma

Lymphocytic leukemia

Myeloproliferative disease

Myeloma

### SOLID TUMORS WITH BONE METASTASIS

Mammary adenocarcinoma

Nasal adenocarcinoma

Epithelial-derived tumors

Pancreatic adenocarcinoma

Lung carcinoma

## SOLID TUMORS WITHOUT BONE METASTASIS

Apocrine gland adenocarcinoma of the anal sac
Interstitial cell tumor
Squamous cell carcinoma
Thyroid adenocarcinoma
Lung carcinoma
Pancreatic adenocarcinoma
Fibrosarcoma

## Lymphoma

## Common Differential Diagnoses

### GENERALIZED LYMPHADENOPATHY

Disseminated infections
- Bacterial, fungal, rickettsial, parasitic, viral
Immune-mediated disease
- SLE, polyarthritis, vasculitis, dermatopathy
Other hematopoietic tumors
- Leukemia, multiple myeloma, malignant or systemic histiocytosis, systemic mastocytosis
Neoplasia metastatic to lymph nodes
Generalized dermatopathy, external parasites
Benign reactive hyperplastic syndromes in cats

### ALIMENTARY DISEASE

Inflammatory bowel diseases
- Lymphocytic/plasmacytic, eosinophilic enteritis
Nonlymphoid intestinal neoplasia
Granulomatous enteritis
Granulated round cell tumors in cats
GI mast cell neoplasia in cats
GI eosinophilic sclerosing fibrosis

### CUTANEOUS DISEASE

Infectious dermatitis (deep pyoderma, fungal dermatitis)
Immune-mediated dermatitis (e.g., PF)
Other cutaneous neoplasms

### MEDIASTINAL DISEASE

Thymoma
Chemodectoma (heart base tumor)
Ectopic thyroid neoplasia
Pulmonary lymphomatoid granulomatosis
Granulomatous disease (e.g., hilar lymphadenopathy with blastomycosis)

## Oral Cavity Tumors, Differential Diagnosis

## Malignant Neoplasms

Melanoma
Squamous cell carcinoma
Fibrosarcoma
Peripheral nerve sheath tumor
Osteosarcoma
Lingual carcinoma or sarcoma
Histiocytic sarcoma
Lymphoma
MCT
Hemangiosarcoma

## Benign Neoplasms

Epulides (acanthomatous ameloblastoma)
- Peripheral odontogenic fibroma (replaces the terms *fibro-matous epulis* and *ossifying epulis*)
- Acanthomatous ameloblastoma (replaces the term *acanthomatous epulis*): may be invasive but does not metastasize
- Giant cell epulis
Papillomas: self-limiting
Fibroma
Lipoma
Chondroma
Osteoma
Odontoma
Cementoma
Plasmacytoma
Hemangioma
Hemangiopericytoma
Histiocytoma
Eosinophilic granuloma
Feline inductive odontogenic tumor

## Skin and Subcutaneous Tumors

### EPITHELIAL TUMORS

Sebaceous gland adenoma/adenocarcinoma
Squamous cell carcinoma
- Canine cutaneous squamous cell carcinoma
- Canine nasal planum squamous cell carcinoma
- Canine digital squamous cell carcinoma
- Canine oral squamous cell carcinoma
- Feline cutaneous squamous cell carcinoma (nasal planum, aural/pinnal, periocular, ear canal)

- Feline oral squamous cell carcinoma
- Feline multicentric squamous cell carcinoma in situ (Bowen disease)

Trichoepithelioma

Intracutaneous cornifying epithelioma

Basal cell tumors

- Benign tumors
- Basal carcinoma

Trichoblastoma

Pilomatricoma

Papilloma

Perianal gland tumors (hepatoid gland tumors)

Sweat gland tumors (apocrine gland tumors)

Ceruminous gland tumors

Anal sac, apocrine gland tumors

Follicular stem cell carcinoma

## ROUND CELL TUMORS

Lymphoma

MCT

Histiocytoma

Transmissible venereal tumor (TVT)

Plasmacytoma

## MESENCHYMAL TUMORS

Soft tissue sarcomas

## MELANOCYTIC TUMORS

Melanoma

- Benign (typically melanomas of haired skin and eyelids)
- Malignant (typically those of digit or mucocutaneous junctions)

## Urogenital Tumors, Classification

### KIDNEY

Lymphoma (most common renal tumor in cats)

Primary renal carcinoma, adenoma/adenocarcinoma

Cystadenocarcinoma with concurrent nodular dermato-fibrosis in German Shepherds

Tumors of embryonic origin (e.g., Wilm tumor)

Nephroblastoma

Transitional cell carcinoma

### URINARY BLADDER

Older female dogs, West Highland White Terriers, Scottish Terriers, Beagles, Dachshunds, Shetland Sheepdogs

Transitional cell carcinoma
Squamous cell carcinoma
Leiomyosarcoma
Leiomyoma
Rhabdomyosarcoma
Metastatic neoplasia
- Hemangiosarcoma
- Lymphoma
- Extension of prostate neoplasia

## PROSTATE
Prostatic adenocarcinoma
Transitional cell carcinoma

## PENIS AND PREPUCE
Prepuce affected by tumors of haired skin seen elsewhere
Penile
- TVT (transmissible venereal tumor)
- Others

## TESTICULAR NEOPLASIA
Cryptorchid dogs are 13.6 times more likely to develop
Sertoli cell tumor or seminoma.
Sertoli cell tumor (25%–50% are functional and cause
hyperestrogenemia)
Leydig cell (interstitial) tumor
Seminoma

## VAGINA AND VULVA
Leiomyoma
Fibroleiomyoma
Fibroma
Polyps
Lipoma
Leiomyosarcoma (rare)
TVT

## UTERUS
Leiomyoma
Leiomyosarcoma
Uterine adenocarcinoma

## OVARY
*Epithelial Tumors (50% of Ovarian Tumors)*
Papillary adenoma
Cystadenoma
Papillary adenocarcinoma
Undifferentiated adenocarcinoma

*Germ Cell Tumors (10% of Ovarian Tumors)*
Dysgerminoma
Teratoma
Teratocarcinoma

*Sex-Cord Stromal Tumors (40% of Ovarian Tumors)*
Granulosa cell tumor
Benign thecoma
Benign luteoma
Sertoli-Leydig cell tumor

### MAMMARY GLAND
Fibroadenoma (mixed mammary tumor)
Solid carcinomas
Tubular adenocarcinoma
Sarcoma
Inflammatory carcinomas
Feline mammary adenocarcinomas

## Paraneoplastic Syndromes

## Classification

### GENERAL
Cancer anorexia, cachexia
Fever

### HEMATOLOGIC
Anemia
- Anemia of chronic disease
- Immune-mediated hemolytic anemia
- Bone marrow infiltration
- Blood loss anemia
- Hyperestrogenism
- Microangiopathic hemolytic anemia

Polycythemia (rare)
- Associated with renal neoplasia, nasal fibrosarcoma, lymphoma, bronchial carcinoma, cecal leiomyosarcoma, transmissible venereal tumor, soft tissue sarcoma

Leukocytosis
- Neutrophilic
- Eosinophilic

Thrombocytopenia
- Increased consumption
- Decreased production (bone marrow neoplasia)
- Increased destruction (immune-mediated thrombocytopenia)

Thrombocytosis
Thrombocyte hyperaggregability/hypercoagulability
Pancytopenia
Coagulation disorders
- DIC
- Coagulation-activating substances produced by tumor
Hyperproteinemia/hyperglobulinemia

## ENDOCRINE

Hypercalcemia of malignancy
Hypoglycemia
Syndrome of inappropriate ADH secretion
- Hyponatremia, serum
- Hypoosmolality, urine
- Hyperosmolality
Hyperestrogenism (Sertoli cell tumor)
Ectopic ACTH

## GASTROINTESTINAL

Gastroduodenal ulceration
- MCTs, gastrinoma
Cancer cachexia

## RENAL

Glomerulonephritis
Hypercalcemic nephropathy

## CUTANEOUS

Superficial necrolytic dermatitis (glucagonoma)
Nodular dermatofibrosis
Feline paraneoplastic alopecia
Flushing (MCT, pheochromocytoma)
Cutaneous necrosis of the hind paws (cats, lymphoma)
Pemphigus vulgaris (dogs, lymphoma)

## NEUROMUSCULAR

Myasthenia gravis
- Dogs with thymoma, osteosarcoma, biliary carcinoma
Peripheral neuropathy
- Multiple myeloma, lymphoma, insulinoma, various carcinomas and sarcomas

## HYPERTROPHIC OSTEOPATHY

Space-occupying mass in thorax or rarely, abdomen

## Sarcomas

### Classification of Soft Tissue Sarcomas

Fibrosarcoma
MCT
Undifferentiated sarcoma
Hemangiosarcoma
Peripheral nerve-sheath tumor(hemangiopericytoma, malignant schwannoma, neurofibroma)
Myxosarcoma
Leiomyosarcoma
Malignant fibrous histiocytoma
Synovial cell sarcoma
Rhabdomyosarcoma
Liposarcoma
Vaccine-associated fibrosarcoma (cats)

### Clinical Findings for Hemangiosarcoma

Older dogs and cats
Many potential sites of origin
- Spleen
- Right atrium
- Subcutis
- Pericardium
- Liver
- Muscle
- Lung
- Skin
- Bone
- Kidney
- CNS
- Peritoneum
- Oral cavity
- Nasal cavity
- Eye
- Retroperitoneum
Hemoabdomen
Pericardial effusion
Cardiac tamponade
Sudden death
Anorexia, vomiting
Lethargy
Right-sided heart failure
Muffled heart sounds
Arrhythmias
Neurologic signs (may metastasize to brain)

## Thyroid Neoplasms

### Classification and Clinical Findings

#### CATS
Hyperthyroidism: functional thyroid tumors
- Thyroid adenoma
- Thyroid adenocarcinoma

#### DOGS
Nonfunctional tumors (90%)
Thyroid adenoma
Thyroid adenocarcinoma
- Swelling or mass in neck
- Dyspnea
- Cough
- Lethargy
- Dysphagia
- Regurgitation
- Anorexia
- Weight loss
- Horner syndrome
- Change in bark/laryngeal paralysis
- Facial edema

Functional tumors (10%)
Thyroid adenoma
Thyroid adenocarcinoma
- Swelling or mass in neck
- Polyphagia/weight
- Hyperactivity
- Polyuria/polydipsia
- Panting
- Change in behavior (aggression)

## Tumors

### Bone and Joint Tumors, Classification

Canine osteosarcoma
- Appendicular
- Skull
- Scapular
- Pelvic
- Ribs
- Vertebral
- Nasal and paranasal

Chondrosarcoma

Fibrosarcoma
Hemangiosarcoma
Multilobular osteochondrosarcoma
Osteoma
Canine multiple cartilaginous exostoses
Feline osteosarcoma
Feline multiple cartilaginous exostoses
Metastatic bone tumors
- Transitional cell carcinoma
- Prostatic adenocarcinoma
- Mammary carcinoma
- Thyroid carcinoma
- Pulmonary carcinoma
- Nasal carcinoma
- Apocrine gland, anal sac adenocarcinoma
- Renal tumors
- Others

Primary joint tumors
- Synovial cell sarcoma
- Histiocytic sarcoma
- Malignant fibrous histiocytoma
- Synovial myxoma
- Myxosarcoma
- Osteosarcoma
- Fibrosarcoma
- Chondrosarcoma
- Hemangiosarcoma
- Liposarcoma
- Rhabdomyosarcoma
- Undifferentiated sarcoma

## Hematopoietic Tumors, Classification

### LYMPHOMA

*Feline*

Alimentary
Multicentric
Mediastinal/thymic
Nasal
Renal
Spinal
Peripheral nodal
Hepatic
CNS
Other
FeLV-associated

*Canine*
Multicentric
Others (alimentary, mediastinal, cutaneous)

## LYMPHOID LEUKEMIA
Acute lymphoblastic leukemia (in cats, often associated with FeLV infection)
Chronic lymphocytic leukemia

## NONLYMPHOID LEUKEMIAS AND MYELOPROLIFERATIVE DISORDERS
Acute myelogenous leukemia (myeloblastic)
Acute myelomonocytic leukemia (myeloblasts/monoblasts)
Acute monocytic leukemia (monoblasts)
Acute megakaryoblastic leukemia (megakaryoblasts)
Erythroleukemia (erythroblasts)

## CHRONIC MYELOPROLIFERATIVE DISORDERS
Chronic myelogenous leukemia (neutrophils, late precursors)
Primary thrombocythemia (platelets)
Basophilic leukemia (basophils and precursors)
Eosinophilic leukemia (eosinophils and precursors)
Polycythemia vera (erythrocytes)
Mast cell leukemia

## PLASMA CELL NEOPLASMS
Multiple myeloma
Solitary plasmacytoma
IgM (Waldenström macroglobulinemia)

## Mast Cell Tumor Disease, Clinical Findings

### CLINICAL APPEARANCE AND LOCATION OF MAST CELL TUMORS
Extremely variable in appearance
Soft, fluctuant, firm, discrete, diffuse, small, large, solitary, multiple, haired, hairless, dermal, or subcutaneous
Erythema, bruising, ulceration
On trunk most often; also perineum, extremities, head, neck
May shrink or swell due to degranulation
Rarely oral cavity, nasal cavity, larynx, conjunctiva

### SYSTEMIC SIGNS OF DISSEMINATED MASTOCYTOSIS
GI ulceration
Abdominal discomfort

Vomiting
Melena
Hypotension
Coagulation abnormalities
Acute or chronic blood loss anemia

# Neurologic and Neuromuscular Disorders

## Brain Disease, Congenital or Hereditary

### Differential Diagnosis

#### CONGENITAL MALFORMATIONS

Failure of normal closure of neural tube: vary in severity from clinically inapparent (agenesis of corpus callosum) to severe (anencephaly)

Lissencephaly: failure of normal migration of neurons in development of cerebral cortex; leads to abnormal appearance of sulci and gyri (most often seen in Lhasa Apsos)

Cerebellar hypoplasia: seen most often in cats after in utero panleukopenia infection; rarely seen with parvovirus infection of developing cerebellum in dogs; may be isolated malformation without infection

Chiari-like malformations: protrusion of cerebellar vermis through foramen magnum (Cavalier King Charles Spaniels, other dog breeds)

Hydrocephalus: congenital hydrocephalus seen most often in toy and brachycephalic breeds; suggests hereditary basis; often congenital stenosis or aplasia of mesencephalic aqueducts

Inborn errors of metabolism (hereditary): young pure-bred animals with diffuse, symmetric signs of brain disease

- Organic acidurias
- Spongiform encephalopathies: may be hereditary or acquired (transmissible) disease
- Polioencephalopathies: metabolic defects that affect gray matter
- Neuroaxonal dystrophy: spheroids causing swelling within axons
- Leukoencephalopathies: disorders of myelin; affect white matter; often affect cerebellum and long tracts, leading to tremors and dysmetria
- Lysosomal storage diseases: accumulation of metabolic products in lysosomes
- Ceroid lipofuscinosis: accumulation of proteins in lysosomes
- Neonatal encephalopathy: hereditary disease of Standard Poodles

## MOVEMENT DISORDERS

Hereditary cerebellar hypoplasia

Multisystem degeneration: diseases of cerebellum and basal ganglia—progressive neuronal abiotrophy of Kerry Blue Terriers and Chinese Crested Dogs

Dyskinesis and dystonias

Paroxysmal dyskinesias ("Scotty cramp" or idiopathic cerebellitis)—Scottish Terriers

## Cognitive Dysfunction

### Clinical Findings

Disorientation

Sleep/wake cycle alterations

House soiling problems

Change in activity levels

- Increased
- Stereotypic
- Decreased

Agitation

Anxiety

Altered responsiveness to stimuli

- Heightened
- Reduced

Changes in appetite

- Increased
- Decreased

Decreased ability to perform learned tasks
Changes in interaction with owners/other pets

## Cranial Nerve Deficits

### Clinical Findings

**CRANIAL NERVE I (OLFACTORY)**
Hyposmia or anosmia

**CRANIAL NERVE II (OPTIC)**
Loss of vision, loss of menace response, dilated pupil, loss of papillary light reflex (direct and consensual)

**CRANIAL NERVE III (OCULOMOTOR)**
Loss of papillary light reflex on affected side (even if light shone in opposite eye), dilated pupil, ptosis, ventrolateral strabismus

**CRANIAL NERVE IV (TROCHLEAR)**
Slight dorsomedial eye rotation

**CRANIAL NERVE V (TRIGEMINAL)**
Atrophy of temporalis and masseter muscles, loss of jaw tone and strength, dropped jaw (if bilateral), analgesia of innervated areas

**CRANIAL NERVE VI (ABDUCENS)**
Medial strabismus, impaired lateral gaze, poor retraction of globe

**CRANIAL NERVE VII (FACIAL)**
Lip, eyelid, and ear droop; loss of ability to blink; loss of ability to retract lip; possibly decreased tear production

**CRANIAL NERVE VIII (VESTIBULOCOCHLEAR)**
Ataxia, head tilt, nystagmus, deafness, positional strabismus

**CRANIAL NERVE IX (GLOSSOPHARYNGEAL)**
Loss of gag reflex, dysphagia

**CRANIAL NERVE X (VAGUS)**
Loss of gag reflex, laryngeal paralysis, dysphagia, megaesophagus

**CRANIAL NERVE XI (ACCESSORY)**
Atrophy of trapezius, sternocephalicus, and brachiocephalicus muscles

### CRANIAL NERVE XII (HYPOGLOSSAL)

Loss of tongue strength, inability to retract tongue if bilateral, atrophy of tongue

## Disorders Confused with Seizures

### Episodic Weakness

Hypoglycemia
Electrolyte disturbances
Low blood cortisol

### Syncope (Decreased Cerebral Blood Flow)

Cardiac arrhythmias
Hypotension

### Myasthenia Gravis

#### ACUTE VESTIBULAR DISEASE

*Exercise-Induced Weakness or Collapse Disorders*
Dynamin-associated exercise induced collapse (dEIC)
Border Collie collapse

*Sleep Disorders*
Narcolepsy
Cataplexy

*Movement Disorders (Dyskinesias)*

## Head Tilt

### Differential Diagnosis

#### PERIPHERAL VESTIBULAR DISEASE

Otitis media/interna
Feline idiopathic vestibular disease
Geriatric canine vestibular disease
Feline nasopharyngeal polyps
Middle ear tumor
- Ceruminous gland adenocarcinoma
- Squamous cell carcinoma

Trauma
Aminoglycoside ototoxicity/chemical ototoxicity
Hypothyroidism (possibly)
Post external ear cleaning/middle ear surgery

#### CENTRAL VESTIBULAR DISEASE

Trauma/hemorrhage
Infectious inflammatory disease
- Rocky Mountain spotted fever
- FIP
- Others

Granulomatous meningoencephalitis, necrotizing
meningoencephalitis
Neoplasia
Vascular infarct
Thiamine deficiency
Metronidazole toxicity
Congenital/developmental
Thiamine deficiency (cats)

## Inflammatory Disease of the Nervous System

### Differential Diagnosis

Steroid-responsive meningitis-arteritis (steroid-responsive
suppurative meningitis) (juvenile to young adult large
breed)
Dogs: Bernese Mountain Dogs, Boxers, German Shorthaired
Pointers, Nova Scotia Duck Tolling Retrievers
Granulomatous meningoencephalitis
- Idiopathic inflammatory brain disease of dogs
- Most commonly in small-breed dogs
Pug meningoencephalitis
- Necrotizing meningoencephalitis of cerebral cortex
- Maltese and Yorkshire Terriers also
Eosinophilic meningoencephalitis
- Idiopathic most frequently (Rottweilers, Golden
Retrievers, Belgian Tervurens, others)
- Secondary to infectious agents (*Cryptococcus neoformans,
Neospora caninum, Baylisascaris procyonis*)
Feline polioencephalomyelitis
- Young cats, progressive course
FIV encephalopathy
Bacterial meningitis and myelitis
- *Staphylococcus aureus*
- *Staphylococcus epidermidis*
- *Staphylococcus albus*
- *Pasteurella multocida*
- *Actinomyces*
- *Nocardia*
- Others
Canine distemper virus
Rabies
FIP
Other viral encephalitides
- Canine herpesvirus
- Feline Borna disease virus
- Pseudorabies virus

- West Nile virus

Toxoplasmosis

Neosporosis

Borreliosis

Mycotic infections

- *Cryptococcus neoformans, C. gattii*
- Other disseminated systemic mycoses

Rickettsial diseases

- Rocky Mountain spotted fever
- Ehrlichiosis
- *Ehrlichia ewingii, Anaplasma phagocytophum*

Parasitic meningitis, myelitis, encephalitis

- Aberrant parasite migration

## Intracranial Neoplasms

### Differential Diagnosis

#### MENINGIOMA
Benign tumor of cells of meninges

#### NEUROEPITHELIAL TUMORS
Gliomas (astrocytomas, oligodendrogliomas)
Choroid plexus tumors (choroid plexus papilloma, choroid plexus carcinoma)
Ependymal tumors
Neuronal and mixed neuronal-glial tumors
Pineal region tumors

#### CENTRAL NERVOUS SYSTEM LYMPHOMA
Primary: neoplasia of native CNS lymphocytes
Secondary: metastasis of systemic lymphoma

#### MESENCHYMAL TUMORS
Lipoma, fibrosarcoma, histiocytoma, leiomyoma, rhabdomyosarcoma, osteosarcoma, others

#### METASTATIC NEOPLASIA TO CENTRAL NERVOUS SYSTEM
Local invasion: nasal adenocarcinoma
Hematogenous spread: melanoma, hemangiosarcoma, lymphosarcoma
Many other neoplasms may metastasize to CNS.

#### PITUITARY TUMORS
Functional tumors of pars distalis or pars intermedius: cause pituitary-dependent hyperadrenocorticism; generally cause little damage to surrounding tissue
Pituitary macrotumor

## Myasthenia Gravis

*Congenital myasthenia gravis:* inherited deficiency of acetylcholine receptors at presynaptic membranes of skeletal muscle

*Acquired myasthenia gravis:* antibodies made against nicotinic acetylcholine receptors of skeletal muscle

### Clinical Findings

Appendicular muscle weakness
- Worsens with exercise
- Improves with rest
- Tetraplegia

Mentation, postural reactions, reflexes normal

Megaesophagus
- Salivation
- Regurgitation (more common in dogs)

Dysphagia

Ventroflexion (more common in cats)

Urinary bladder distension

Hoarse bark or meow

Persistently dilated pupils

Facial muscle weakness

Aspiration pneumonia

Respiratory weakness

## Myositis and Myopathies

### Differential Diagnosis

#### INFLAMMATORY MYOPATHIES

Masticatory myositis
- IgG antibodies to type 2M myofibers
- German Shepherds, Retrievers, Cavalier King Charles Spaniels, and Doberman Pinschers predisposed
- Young to middle-aged dogs

Canine immune-mediated polymyositis
- Large-breed dogs predisposed

Feline immune-mediated polymyositis

Dermatomyositis
- Herding breeds, especially Shetland Sheepdogs and Collies

Protozoal myositis
- *Toxoplasma gondii*
- *Neospora caninum, Hepatozoon, Babesia, Leishmania,* or *Trypanosoma* infection

Bacterial myositis
- *Clostridium, Leptospira, Ehrlichia,* Rocky Mountain spotted fever

Extraocular myositis (dogs)

FIV

## METABOLIC MYOPATHIES

Glucocorticoid excess
- Hyperadrenocorticism
- Exogenous corticosteroids

Hypothyroidism

Hypoadrenocorticism

Hypokalemic polymyopathy (cat)
- Increased urinary excretion
- Decreased dietary intake

Mitochondrial myopathies

Lipid storage myopathies

Glycogen storage disorders

Malignant hyperthermia

Hyperkalemic periodic paralysis (American Pit Bull Terrier)

## INHERITED MYOPATHIES

Muscular dystrophies
- Hereditary Golden Retriever muscular dystrophy
- Also German Shorthaired Pointer, Rottweiler, others
- Maine Coon, Siamese, Devon Rex, Sphinx, others

Myotonia—Chow Chow, Staffordshire Bull Terrier, Labrador Retriever, Rhodesian Ridgeback, Great Dane, others

Malignant hyperthermia
- Hypermetabolic disorder of skeletal muscle
- Genetic defect in intracellular calcium homeostasis

Inherited myopathy of Great Danes

Centronuclear myopathy—Labrador Retriever

Episodic/exercise-induced collapse—Labrador Retriever

Exertional rhabdomyolysis

## Neurologic Examination

### Components

#### MENTAL STATE

Normal

Depression/lethargy

Stupor

Coma

Agitation

Delirium

## POSTURE
Normal, upright
Head tilt
Tremor
Wide-based stance
Plantigrade stance
Recumbent
Extensor posturing
Opisthotonus
Pleurothotonus

## GAIT
Proprioceptive deficits
Paresis
Circling
Ataxia
Dysmetria
Lameness

## POSTURAL REACTIONS
Conscious proprioception
Hopping
Wheelbarrowing
Paw placement
Hemiwalking
Extensor postural thrust

## MUSCLE TONE
Atrophy
Decreased muscle tone (lesions of lower motor neurons)
Increased muscle tone (lesions of upper motor neurons)
Schiff-Sherrington posture (increased muscle tone and
    hyperextension of thoracic limbs)

## SPINAL REFLEXES
Absent, depressed, normal, or exaggerated
Thoracic limb withdrawal (sixth cervical [C6], C7, C8,
    first thoracic [T1])
Biceps (C6–C8) and triceps (C7–T2) reflexes
Patellar (fourth lumbar [L4], L5, L6)
Pelvic limb withdrawal (L6, L7, first sacral [S1])
Sciatic (L6, L7, S1)
Cranial tibial (L6, L7)
Perineal (S1, S2, S3, pudendal nerve)
Bulbourethral (S1, S2, S3, pudendal nerve)
Panniculus (response absent caudal to spinal cord lesion,
    used at T3–L3)
Crossed extensor reflex (indicative of upper motor neu-
    ron [UMN] disease)
Cutaneous trunci reflex

### SENSATION AND PAIN
Superficial pain
Deep pain
Hyperesthesia

### URINARY TRACT FUNCTION

### CRANIAL NERVES

## Paroxysmal Disorders Confused With Epileptic Seizures

### Differential Diagnosis

#### SYNCOPE (REDUCED CEREBRAL BLOOD FLOW)
Cardiac arrhythmias
Hypotension

#### EPISODIC WEAKNESS
Hypoglycemia
Low blood cortisol
Electrolyte disturbances

#### MYASTHENIA GRAVIS

#### ACUTE VESTIBULAR EPISODES

#### MOVEMENT DISORDERS
Episodic falling
Scotty cramp
Head bobbing
Dyskinesias

#### SLEEP DISORDERS
Narcolepsy
Cataplexy

#### OBSESSIVE-COMPULSIVE DISORDER

## Peripheral Neuropathies

Clinical signs depend on the nerve affected and the severity of the lesion.

### Differential Diagnosis

#### FOCAL DISEASE
*Trauma*
Mechanical blows
Fractures
Pressure
Stretching

Laceration
Injection of agents into nerves

*Peripheral Nerve Tumors*
Schwannoma
Neurofibroma
Neurofibrosarcoma
Lymphoma

*Facial Nerve Paralysis*
Otitis media
Trauma
Neoplasia
Foreign body (e.g., grass awn)
Nasopharyngeal polyp in cats
Hypothyroidism
Idiopathic

*Trigeminal Nerve Paralysis*
Bilateral, idiopathic disorder, often self-limiting
Middle-aged to older dogs, rarely cats

*Idiopathic Peripheral Vestibular Disease*
Brachial plexus neuritis

*Hyperchylomicronemia*
Leads to xanthomas in skin
May compress peripheral nerves

*Ischemic Neuromyopathy*
Caudal aortic thromboembolism

## GENERALIZED CHRONIC POLYNEUROPATHIES
Idiopathic
Metabolic disorders
- Diabetes mellitus
- Hypothyroidism
Paraneoplastic syndromes
- Insulinoma
- Other tumors
SLE or other immune-mediated disease
Chronic organophosphate toxicity
Ehrlichiosis

## GENERALIZED ACUTE NEUROPATHIES
Acute polyradiculoneuritis ("Coonhound paralysis")
Neospora polyradiculoneuritis (puppies)
Disorders of neuromuscular junction
- Botulism
- Tick paralysis
- Myasthenia gravis

Protozoal polyradiculoneuritis

Toxins

Dysautonomia

## DEVELOPMENTAL/CONGENITAL NEUROPATHIES

Loss of motor neurons—Cairn Terrier, German Shepherd, English Pointer, Rottweiler, Swedish Lapland, Brittany Spaniel

Loss of peripheral axons—German Shepherd, Alaskan Malamute, Birman cat, Rottweiler, Boxer, Dalmatian

Schwann cell dysfunction—Golden Retriever, Tibetan Mastiff

Loss of sensory neuron of axon and laryngeal nerves— Dachshund, English Pointer, Shorthaired Pointer, Bouvier des Flandres, Siberian Husky

Inborn errors of metabolism

- Hyperchylomicronemia (cat)
- Hyperoxaluria type 2 (shorthaired cat)
- α-L-fucosidosis (English Springer Spaniel)
- Atypical GM2 gangliosidosis (cat)
- Globoid cell leukodystrophy
- Niemann–Pick disease (Siamese)
- Glycogen storage disease (Norwegian Forest Cat)

## Spinal Cord Disease

## Differential Diagnosis

### ACUTE

Trauma

Hemorrhage/coagulopathy

Infarction

Type I intervertebral disk herniation

Fibrocartilaginous embolism

Atlantoaxial subluxation

### SUBACUTE/PROGRESSIVE

Discospondylitis

Noninfectious inflammatory diseases

- Corticosteroid-responsive meningitis/arteritis
- Granulomatous meningoencephalitis
- Feline polioencephalomyelitis

Infectious inflammatory diseases

- Bacterial, fungal, rickettsial, protothecal, protozoal, nematodiasis

Distemper myelitis

FIP meningitis/myelitis

## CHRONIC PROGRESSIVE
Neoplasia
Type II intervertebral disk protrusion
Degenerative myelopathy
Degenerative lumbosacral stenosis (cauda equina syndrome)
Cervical spondylomyelopathy (vertebral malformation/malarticulation, wobbler syndrome)
Lumbosacral vertebral canal stenosis
Spondylosis deformans
Hypervitaminosis A (cats)
Dural ossification
Diffuse idiopathic skeletal hyperostosis
Synovial cyst

## PROGRESSIVE IN YOUNG ANIMALS
Neuronal abiotrophies and degenerations
Metabolic storage diseases
Atlantoaxial luxation
Congenital vertebral anomalies

## CONGENITAL (CONSTANT)
Spinal bifida
Congenital dysgenesis of Manx cats
Spinal dysraphism
Hereditary ataxia
Pilonidal, epidermoid, and dermoid cysts
Syringomyelia/hydromyelia

## Spinal Cord Lesions

### Localization

## CRANIAL CERVICAL LESION (C1–C5)
UMN signs in hindlimbs
UMN signs in forelimbs

## CAUDAL CERVICAL LESION (C6–T2)
UMN signs in hindlimbs
Lower motor neuron (LMN) signs in forelimbs

## THORACOLUMBAR LESION (T3–L3)
UMN signs in hindlimbs
Normal forelimbs

## LUMBOSACRAL LESION (L4–S3)
LMN signs in hindlimbs
Loss of perineal sensation and reflexes
Normal forelimbs

### SACRAL LESION (S1–S3)
Normal forelimbs
Normal patellar reflexes
Loss of sciatic function
Loss of perineal sensation and reflexes

## Systemic Disease

## Neurologic Manifestations

### OXYGEN DEPRIVATION

*Vascular Disease*

Ischemia
Thromboembolic disease
Shock
Cardiac disease

Hemorrhage (Anemia)
Vessel rupture secondary to hypertension
Coagulopathy
Vasculitis

*Anesthetic Accidents (Hypotension, Cardiac Arrhythmia, Extensive Blood Loss, Hypercapnia, Hypoxemia)*

*Hypoxia*
Pulmonary disease
Decreased oxygen transport
Heart failure

*Hypertension*

### HYPOGLYCEMIA

*Decreased Output or Metabolism*
Primary liver disease
Malnutrition
Thiamine deficiency

*Increased Uptake*
Hyperinsulinemia
Islet cell tumors
Insulin overdose

Non–Islet Cell Neoplasia
Hepatoma
Leiomyoma

Excessive Metabolism
Sepsis
Breed- or activity-related

*Increased Uptake of Amino Acids by Extrahepatic Tissues*

## WATER AND IONIC IMBALANCES

*Water*

Hypoosmolar States (Retention of Free Water)
Hyponatremia

Hyperosmolar States (Loss of Free Water)
Hypernatremia (diabetes insipidus)
Hyperglycemia (diabetes mellitus)

Ions (Excess or Deficiency)
Calcium
Potassium

## ENDOGENOUS NEUROTOXINS

*Renal Toxins*

*Hepatoencephalopathy*

*Endocrine Disease*

Adrenal
Hyperadrenocorticism
Hypoadrenocorticism

Adrenergic Dysregulation
Pheochromocytoma

Thyroid
Hypothyroidism
• Myxedema
• Neuromyopathy
Thyrotoxicosis
• Hyperthyroidism
• Iatrogenic

## EXOGENOUS NEUROTOXINS

Plant toxins
Sedative depressant drugs (e.g., antiepileptic drugs)
Heat stroke

## REMOTE NEUROLOGIC MANIFESTATIONS OF CANCER

Metastasis to the nervous system
Vascular accidents and infection
Adverse effects of therapy
Paraneoplastic syndromes

## Vestibular Disease

### Clinical Findings

#### CENTRAL AND PERIPHERAL VESTIBULAR DISEASE

Head tilt to side of lesion
Circling/falling/rolling to side of lesion
Vomiting, salivation
Incoordination
Ventral strabismus on side of lesion (±)
Nystagmus, fast-phase away from lesion
Nystagmus may intensify with changes in body position.

#### PERIPHERAL VESTIBULAR DISEASE

Nystagmus is horizontal or rotatory.
No change in nystagmus direction with changes in head position
Postural reactions and proprioception normal
Concurrent Horner syndrome, CN VII paralysis with middle/inner ear involvement; other CNs normal

#### CENTRAL VESTIBULAR DISEASE

Nystagmus horizontal, rotatory, or vertical
Nystagmus direction may change direction with change in head position
Abnormal postural reactions and proprioception may be seen on side of lesion
Multiple CN deficits may be seen

#### PARADOXICAL VESTIBULAR SYNDROME (CEREBELLAR LESION)

Head tilt and circling away from side of lesion
Fast-phase nystagmus toward the lesion
May exhibit vertical nystagmus
Abnormal postural reactions on side of lesion
± Multiple cranial nerve deficits on side of lesion
± Hypermetria, truncal sway, and head tremor

# Ocular Disorders

## Anisocoria

### Differential Diagnosis

#### NONNEUROLOGIC CAUSES OF ANISOCORIA

*Conditions That Cause Miosis*
Anterior uveitis
Corneal ulcers and lacerations (reflex miosis mediated by trigeminal nerve)

*Conditions That Cause Mydriasis*
Iris atrophy
Iris coloboma
Iris hypoplasia
Glaucoma
Iridal tumors (e.g., melanoma) that infiltrate iridal musculature
Unilateral retinal disease (e.g., retinal detachment)
Severe chorioretinitis that affects a larger area on one eye than the other
Unilateral optic neuritis or optic nerve neoplasia
Orbital neoplasia, retrobulbar abscess, cellulitis

*Pharmacologic Causes of Anisocoria*
Drugs that Cause Miosis (usually agents used for management of glaucoma)
Pilocarpine
Demecarium bromide
Synthetic prostaglandins such as latanoprost

Drugs That Cause Mydriasis
Tropicamide, atropine

Ocular contact with toxins like jimsonweed
*(Datura stramonium)*
Ocular decongestants like phenylephrine

### *Neurologic Causes of Anisocoria*

#### Afferent Lesions

Anisocoria is reduced or abolished in darkness as
both pupils dilate. This is because the stimulus
producing the anisocoria, light causing constriction of the normal pupil, is eliminated.

- Unilateral retinal or prechiasmal optic nerve
  lesion
- Unilateral optic tract lesion
- Optic chiasm lesion

#### Efferent Lesions

Parasympathetic efferent lesions. (In dogs, preganglionic efferent nerves are purely parasympathetic and postganglionic nerves are mixed. In
cats, both nerves are purely parasympathetic.)

- Lesions of the nucleus of CN III, the preganglionic fibers, or the ganglion itself

Sympathetic efferent lesions. (Loss of sympathetic
tone to the eye is known as *Horner syndrome;*
is always ipsilateral to the lesion; and features
miosis, ptosis, protrusion of the third eyelid, and
enophthalmos.)

- Head, neck, or chest trauma
- Brachial plexus avulsion
- Intracranial, mediastinal, or intrathoracic
  neoplasia
- Otitis media/interna
- Injury to the ear during ear flushing
- Idiopathic (Golden Retrievers and Collies may
  be predisposed)

## Blindness, Acute

## Differential Diagnosis, Dogs and Cats

### CORNEA

Edema (glaucoma, trauma, endothelial dystrophy,
immune-mediated keratitis, neurotropic keratitis,
anterior uveitis)
Melanin (entropion, ectropion, lagophthalmos, facial
nerve paralysis, keratoconjunctivitis sicca, pannus)
Cellular infiltrate (bacterial, viral, fungal)

Vascular invasion (exposure keratitis)
Fibrosis (scar formation)
Dystrophy (lipid, genetic)
Symblepharon (conjunctiva adhered to cornea)

## AQUEOUS HUMOR

Fibrin (anterior uveitis: many etiologies)
Hyphema (trauma, coagulopathies, neoplasia, systemic hypertension, retinal detachment)
Hypopyon (immune-mediated, lymphoma, systemic fungal infection, toxoplasmosis, FIP, protothecosis, brucellosis, bacterial septicemia)
Lipemic (hyperlipidemia with concurrent blood–aqueous barrier disruption [uveitis])

## LENS

Cataracts (genetic, diabetes, retinal degeneration, hypo-calcemia, electric shock, chronic uveitis, lens luxation, metabolic, toxic, traumatic, nutritional)

## VITREOUS

Hemorrhage (trauma, systemic hypertension, retinal detachment, neoplasia, coagulopathy)
Hyalitis (numerous infectious agents, penetrating injury)

## RETINA

Retinopathy (glaucoma, sudden acquired retinal degen-eration [SARD], progressive retinal atrophy, central progressive retinal atrophy, feline central retinal atrophy, toxicity, taurine deficiency in cats, vitamin E deficiency in dogs, enrofloxacin toxicity in cats)
Chorioretinitis (systemic mycoses, ehrlichiosis, Rocky Mountain spotted fever, canine distemper, toxo-plasmosis, FIP, protothecosis, brucellosis, bacterial septicemia, intraocular larval migrans, neoplasia)
Retinal detachment (neoplasia, retinal dysplasia, heredi-tary/congenital, exudative/transudative disorders such as systemic hypertension or infection-induced inflam-matory disease)

## LESIONS THAT PREVENT TRANSMISSION OF THE IMAGE (OPTIC NERVE DISEASE)

Viruses (canine distemper, FIP)
Systemic diseases (neoplasia, traumatic avulsion of optic nerve, granulomatous meningoencephalitis, hydro-cephalus, optic nerve hypoplasia, immune-mediated optic neuritis, systemic mycoses)

### LESIONS THAT PREVENT INTERPRETATION OF THE VISUAL MESSAGE

Canine distemper, FIP, toxoplasmosis, granulomatous meningoencephalitis, systemic mycoses, trauma, heat stroke, hypoxia, hydrocephalus, hepatoencephalopathy, neoplasia, storage diseases, postictal, meningitis

## Corneal Color Changes

### Diagnostic Tests

#### RED (BLOOD VESSELS)

Mechanism is chronic irritation.

Fluorescein stain, Schirmer tear test (STT), palpebral and corneal reflexes

#### "FLUFFY" BLUE (STROMAL EDEMA)

Mechanisms are endothelial or epithelial dysfunction.

Fluorescein stain, intraocular pressure (IOP), flare, check for lens luxation

#### "WISPY" GRAY (STROMAL SCAR)

Mechanism is previous (inactive) inflammation.

Fluorescein stain

#### "SPARKLY" WHITE (LIPID/MINERAL ACCUMULATION)

Mechanisms are dystrophy, degeneration, or hyperlipidemia.

Fluorescein stain, systemic lipid analysis

#### BLACK (PIGMENTATION)

Mechanism is chronic irritation.

Fluorescein stain, STT

#### "PUNCTATE" TAN (KERATINIC PRECIPITATES OR STAPHYLOMA)

Mechanism is uveitis.

IOP, flare, systemic disease testing

#### YELLOW-GREEN (INFLAMMATORY CELL INFILTRATION)

Inflammation (usually septic)

Fluorescein stain, cytology, culture and sensitivity testing, PCR

## Eyelids and Periocular Skin

### Differential Diagnosis

#### INFECTIOUS BLEPHARITIS

*Bacterial Blepharitis*

Usually *Staphylococcus* spp.

External hordeolum or stye—infection of the glands of Zeis or Moll

Internal hordeolum—infection of the meibomian glands

Chalazion—meibomian secretions thicken and obstruct the duct, leading to glandular rupture and lipogranuloma formation

*Fungal Blepharitis*

Dermatophytes (*Microsporum canis, Microsporum gypseum, Trichophyton mentagrophytes*)

*Malassezia pachydermatitis*—most dogs with *Malassezia* dermatitis have concurrent dermatoses; in cats, *Malassezia* infection is linked to systemic disease like diabetes, retroviral infection, internal neoplasia

*Parasitic Blepharitis*

Demodicosis

Feline herpetic ulcerative dermatitis

*Allergic Blepharitis*

Atopic dermatitis

Cutaneous adverse food reaction (food allergy)

*Metabolic/Nutritional Blepharitis*

Zinc-responsive dermatosis

Superficial necrolytic dermatitis (hepatocutaneous disease)

*Immune-Mediated Blepharitis*

PF

PE

SLE

Erythema multiforme

*Iatrogenic Blepharitis (Adverse Reactions to Topical Medications)*

*Pigmentary Changes Involving the Eyelid*

Lentigo simplex of orange cats (black macules, not pathogenic)

Vitiligo (hypopigmentation)

Uveodermatologic (Vogt-Koyanagi-Harada-like) syndrome (leukoderma)

*Neoplastic Blepharitis*

Meibomian gland adenoma

Papillomas

Squamous cell carcinoma

Lymphosarcoma
MCT

*Miscellaneous Eyelid Diseases*
Juvenile sterile granulomatous dermatitis and lymph-
adenitis/juvenile cellulitis (puppy strangles)
Canine reactive histiocytosis
Entropion
Ectropion
Distichiasis
Trichiasis

## Nonhealing Corneal Erosions (Ulcers) in Dogs

### Causes

Establish underlying cause of impaired wound healing
- Mechanical trauma from lid masses
- Entropion, ectropion
- Foreign bodies
- Secondary infection
- Corneal exposure caused by lid paralysis
- Exophthalmos
- Buphthalmos
- Tear film abnormalities
- Conformational abnormalities resulting in
  lagophthalmos
- Corneal edema
- Distichiasis, ectopic cilia
- Facial fold irritation of cornea

#### SPONTANEOUS CHRONIC CORNEAL EPITHELIAL DEFECTS (SCCEDS)—ALSO CALLED *INDOLENT EROSIONS/ULCERS* OR *BOXER EROSIONS/ULCERS*

Middle-aged dogs
Boxers predisposed
Likely instigated by superficial trauma
Dogs with diabetes mellitus predisposed
Rim of loose epithelium surrounds corneal defect
No loss of stromal substance (stromal loss indicates more
severe process, typically infection)
Blepharospasm/epiphora
Neovascularization may be delayed compared with heal-
ing corneal ulcers

#### BULLOUS KERATOPATHY

## Ocular Manifestations of Systemic Diseases

## Surface Ocular Disease

### EYELIDS

Immunosuppressive disorders may predispose to meibomian gland infection with *Demodex* or *Staphylococcus* spp.

Eyelids have mucocutaneous junction; affected by autoimmune disorders such as SLE and pemphigoid diseases; also may be affected by uveodermatologic syndrome and vasculitis

Altered lid position, CN III or VII dysfunction

Horner syndrome: decreased sympathetic tone causing enophthalmos with third eyelid protrusion, ptosis, and miosis; often idiopathic; may be seen with disease of brain, spinal cord, brachial plexus, thorax, mediastinum, neck, temporal bone, tympanic bulla, or orbit

### CONJUNCTIVITIS

May reflect disease of deeper ocular structures

Good location to detect pallor, cyanosis, icterus

Feline herpesvirus type 1 (FHV-1) and *Chlamydophila felis* are primary pathogens of the conjunctiva.

### CORNEA/SCLERA

Creamy pink discoloration of cornea may be seen with lymphoma.

Corneal lipidosis appears similar; it may be secondary to hyperlipidemia from hypothyroidism, hyperadrenocorticism, diabetes mellitus, and familial hypertriglyceridemia.

### KERATOCONJUNCTIVITIS SICCA

Most cases are caused by lymphoplasmacytic dacryoadenitis

Rarely seen with xerostomia (Sjögren-like syndrome)

Possible causes include drug therapy, atropine, sulfa drugs, etodolac, and anesthetic agents.

Others causes include canine distemper, FHV-1, and dysautonomia.

## Uveal Tract, Lens, Fundus

### UVEAL TRACT

*Hyphema or Hemorrhage*

Hypertension, rickettsial disease, trauma, coagulopathy, lymphoma, metastatic neoplasia

*Protein or Fibrin Deposition*
Trauma, FIP, uveodermatologic syndrome, lens capsule rupture, rickettsial disease

*Cellular (Hypopyon) or Granulomatous Infiltrates*
Trauma, lymphoma, metastatic neoplasia, uveodermatologic syndrome, algae or yeast, lens capsule rupture, FIP, systemic mycoses, toxoplasmosis
Other infectious agents associated with uveal tract disease include FIV, FeLV, mycobacteria, FHV-1, *Bartonella* spp., *Ehrlichia* spp., *Leishmania donovani*, *Rickettsia rickettsii*, *Brucella canis*, *Leptospira* spp., and canine adenovirus

*Iris Abnormalities (Papillary Changes)*
Anisocoria with FeLV
Miosis with Horner syndrome
Mydriasis with dysautonomia

## LENS

*Cataracts*
Most common cause in dogs is hereditary.
Cataracts are a frequent complication of diabetes mellitus.
Uveitis may also cause cataracts (most common cause in cats).
Other causes include hypocalcemia (hypoparathyroidism), electric shock, lightning strike, altered nutrition (e.g., puppies fed milk replacer).

*Lens Luxation/Subluxation*
Most often secondary to severe intraocular disease (uveitis)
May be primary in Terriers

## FUNDUS

Usually affected by diseases that extend from the uveal tract (see Uveal Tract p. 277) or from CNS (immune-mediated diseases such as granulomatous meningoencephalitis or neoplasia of CNS)

*Papilledema*
Optic nerve edema without hemorrhage, exudates, or blindness
Seen with increased intracranial pressure

*Taurine Deficiency*
Retinal degeneration
May also cause dilated cardiomyopathy

*Retinal Visualization*
Allows assessment of systemic condition, including anemia (attenuated, pale vessels), hyperlipidemia (creamy orange hue to vessels), and hyperviscosity (increased vessel tortuosity)

*Systemic Hypertension*
Causes extravasation of blood into retina, choroid, or subretinal space

## Ocular Neoplasia

### Orbital Neoplasia (Presents as Exophthalmos, Strabismus, Protrusion of the Third Eyelid, Epiphora, and Exposure Keratitis)

Osteosarcoma
Multilobular osteosarcoma
Fibrosarcoma
Invasion of orbit by neoplasms of surrounding structures such as nose, sinuses, oral cavity, and orbital glands (nasal adenocarcinoma most commonly)
Cats are more likely to have invasion of orbit from surrounding structures (fibrosarcoma, undifferentiated sarcoma, adenocarcinoma, lymphoma); rarely see primary orbital neoplasia (squamous cell carcinoma, melanoma).

### Adnexal Neoplasia (Eyelid Neoplasia Common in Dogs and Rare in Cats)

Some 90% of eyelid tumors are benign (meibomian adenomas, melanomas, papillomas most commonly).
Less common adnexal tumors include histiocytoma, malignant melanoma, adenocarcinoma, basal cell carcinoma, MCT, squamous cell carcinoma, hemangiosarcoma.
Squamous cell carcinoma is the most common eyelid tumor in cats; associated with sun exposure in cats that lack periocular pigmentation.

### Surface Ocular Neoplasia (Tumors of the Conjunctiva, Third Eyelid, Cornea)

Dermoid
Epibulbar or limbal melanocytoma
Conjunctival neoplasia: hemangioma, hemangiosarcoma, MCT, lymphoma, squamous cell carcinoma, papilloma
Third eyelid neoplasia: adenocarcinoma (most common), hemangiosarcoma, lobular adenoma, squamous cell carcinoma, melanoma

## Intraocular Neoplasia (Present With Glaucoma, Hyphema, Corneal Edema, Buphthalmos, Dyscoria, Uveitis, Retinal Detachment, Blindness)

Anterior uveal melanoma (most common); 82% are benign in dogs, poorer prognosis in cats

Other primary tumors of dogs include ciliary body adenocarcinoma and medulloepithelioma.

Other primary tumors of cats include posttraumatic sarcoma and lymphoma.

## Red Eye

### Differential Diagnosis

#### ERYTHEMA OF PRIMARILY CONJUNCTIVAL VESSELS

Corneal ulceration
Eyelid abnormalities
Dacryocystitis
Cilia abnormalities
Keratoconjunctivitis sicca
Allergic conjunctivitis
Bacterial or fungal keratitis
Orbital disease

#### ERYTHEMA OF PRIMARILY EPISCLERAL VESSELS

Anterior uveitis (low IOP)
Glaucoma (high IOP)

#### FOCAL ERYTHEMA

*Masses*

Prolapse of the gland of the third eyelid
Neoplasia
Episcleritis
Nodular granulomatous episcleritis
Granulation tissue

*Hemorrhage*
- Trauma
- Systemic disease (vasculitis, coagulopathy)

## Retinal Detachment

### Differential Diagnosis

#### THREE MAIN MECHANISMS—EXUDATIVE, ASSOCIATED WITH RETINAL TEARS (RHEGMATOGENOUS), OR TRACTION PULLING ON RETINA

Trauma—penetrating injuries such as animal bites, projectiles, or foreign bodies may result in retinal tears or induce intraocular hemorrhage, inflammation, or vitreous infection with subsequent traction retinal detachment. Typically unilateral, although strangulation can lead to bilateral retinal detachment.

Ocular anomalies such as severe retinal dysplasia, optic nerve colobomas, vitreous abnormalities, and retinal nonattachment (developmental failure of the two retinal layers to unite)

Later-onset ocular anomalies such as cataracts and vitreous degeneration may lead to rhegmatogenous retinal detachment, especially with rapid-forming or hypermature cataracts that lead to lens-induced uveitis.

Hypertension is most often related to renal disease but may also be seen with hyperthyroidism and pheochromocytoma.

Hyperviscosity—severe hyperlipidemia, hyperglobulinemia, polycythemia

Neoplasia—most commonly due to multiple myeloma (hyperproteinemia and hyperviscosity) and lymphoma (infiltration of retina and choroid). Large intraocular tumors may induce traction retinal detachment.

Chorioretinitis, retinochoroiditis

Bacteria (leptospirosis, brucellosis, bartonellosis)

Rickettsia (ehrlichiosis, Rocky Mountain spotted fever)

Fungal (aspergillosis, blastomycosis, coccidioidomycosis, histoplasmosis, cryptococcosis)

- Algae (geotrichosis, protot/hecosis)
- Viral (canine distemper virus, FIP)
- Secondary to retroviral infection (FeLV, FIV by predisposing to lymphosarcoma or an opportunistic infection like toxoplasmosis)
- Parasitic (causes smaller areas of detachment—larval migrans of strongyles, ascarids, or *Baylisascaris* larvae, toxoplasmosis, leishmaniasis, neospora, babesiosis)

Immune-mediated disease—causes vasculitis with or without chorioretinitis

- SLE
- Uveodermatologic syndrome
- Granulomatous meningoencephalitis

Toxic—trimethoprim/sulfa or ethylene glycol in dogs, griseofulvin in cats

Idiopathic

## Uveitis

## Differential Diagnosis in the Dog (d) and Cat (c)

### SYSTEMIC INFECTION

*Bacterial*

Bacteremia or septicemia (d, c)

Bartonellosis (d, c)

Leptospirosis (d)

Borreliosis (d)

Brucellosis (d)

*Rickettsial*

Ehrlichiosis (d, c)

Rocky Mountain spotted fever (d)

*Viral*

Canine adenovirus-1 (d)

FeLV (c)

FIV (c)

FIP (c)

*Mycotic*

Blastomycosis (d, c)

Histoplasmosis (d, c)

Coccidiomycosis (d, c)

Cryptomycosis (d, c)

Aspergillosis (d)

*Algal*

Prototheosis (d, c)

*Parasitic*

Aberrant nematode larval migration

*Toxocara* (ocular larval migrans) (d, c)

*Dirofilaria* larvae (d)

*Protozoan*

Toxoplasmosis (d, c)

Leishmaniasis (d, c)

*Immune-Mediated Uveitis*

Idiopathic anterior uveitis (d, c)

Lens-induced uveitis (d, c)

Canine adenovirus vaccine reaction (d)

Uveodermatologic syndrome (d) (primarily Akitas and Arctic breeds)

Pigmentary uveitis (d) (primarily Golden Retrievers)

*Neoplasia*
    Primary (d, c)
    Metastatic (most commonly lymphoma) (d, c)

*Metabolic*
    Diabetes mellitus (lens-induced uveitis) (d)
    Hyperlipidemia (d)

*Trauma*
    Blunt or sharp (d, c)

*Miscellaneous Causes of Blood–Eye Barrier*
 *Disruption*
    Hyperviscosity syndrome (d, c)
    Hypertension (d, c)
    Scleritis (d)
    Ulcerative keratitis (d, c)

# Toxicology

Chemical Toxicoses
Plant Toxicoses
Venomous Bites and Stings

## Chemical Toxicoses

### Toxicants

**KEROSENE, GASOLINE, MINERAL SEAL OIL, TURPENTINE, OTHERS**

Pulmonary, CNS, and GI signs: may lead to hepatotoxicity, renal toxicity, and cardiac arrhythmias

**NAPHTHALENE (MOTHBALLS)**

Vomiting, lethargy, seizures, acute Heinz body hemolytic anemia, methemoglobinemia, hemoglobinuria, renal failure

**ETHANOL, METHANOL (WOOD ALCOHOL)**

CNS depression, behavioral changes, ataxia, hypothermia, respiratory and cardiac arrest

**ETHYLENE GLYCOL**

Early intoxication: ataxia, progresses to oliguric renal failure with renomegaly, vomiting, hypothermia, coma, and death

**SOAPS AND DETERGENTS**

GI irritants

**HOUSEHOLD CORROSIVES**

Toilet bowl cleansers, calcium/lime/rust removers, drain cleaners, oven cleaners, bleaches

**PROPYLENE GLYCOL**

Ataxia, CNS depression

**PHENOL PRODUCTS (HOUSEHOLD CLEANERS)**

Cats particularly sensitive; hepatic and renal damage, ataxia, weakness, tremors, coma, seizures, respiratory alkalosis

**ANTICOAGULANT RODENTICIDES**

Petechiae, ecchymosis, weakness, pallor, respiratory distress, CNS depression, hematemesis, epistaxis, melena, ataxia, paresis, seizures, sudden death

## ZINC PHOSPHATE

Anorexia, lethargy, weakness, abdominal pain, vomiting early after ingestion; progresses to recumbency, tremors, seizures, cardiopulmonary collapse, death

## CHOLECALCIFEROL (VITAMIN D) RODENTICIDES AND MEDICATIONS

Anorexia, CNS depression, vomiting, muscle weakness, constipation, bloody diarrhea, polyuria/polydipsia

## BROMETHALIN RODENTICIDES

High-dose exposure: muscle tremors, hyperexcitability, vocalization, seizures, hyperesthesia, vomiting, dyspnea

## PYRETHRIN AND PYRETHROID INSECTICIDES

CNS depression, hypersalivation, muscle tremors, vomiting, ataxia, dyspnea, anorexia, hypothermia, hyperthermia, seizures, rarely death

## ORGANOPHOSPHATE AND CARBAMATE INSECTICIDES

Muscarinic signs (salivation, lacrimation, bronchial secretion, vomiting, diarrhea) and nicotinic signs (muscle tremors, respiratory paralysis), mixed signs (CNS depression, seizures, miosis, hyperactivity)

## 2,4-DICHLOROPHENOXYACETIC ACID

Vomiting, diarrhea; greater exposure may cause CNS depression, ataxia, and hindlimb myotonia

## LEAD (PAINTS, BATTERIES, LINOLEUM, SOLDER, PLUMBING SUPPLIES, FISHING WEIGHTS)

High-level exposure: vomiting, abdominal pain, anorexia, diarrhea, megaesophagus

CNS signs, behavioral changes, hysteria, ataxia, tremors, opisthotonos, blindness, seizures

## ZINC

Acute ingestion: vomiting, CNS depression, lethargy, diarrhea

Chronic exposure: anorexia, vomiting, diarrhea, CNS depression, pica, hemolysis, regenerative anemia, spherocytosis, inflammatory leukogram, icterus, renal failure

## IRON

Vomiting, diarrhea, abdominal pain, hematemesis, melena; rarely, progresses to multisystemic failure

## Plant Toxicoses

## Plants That Cause Hemolysis

Onion

## Plants That Affect the Cardiovascular System

Cardiac glycoside toxicity: bradycardia with first-, second-, or third-degree AV block, ventricular arrhythmias, asystole, and sudden death; also see GI signs

Common oleander (*Nerium oleander*)

Yellow oleander (*Thevetia peruviana*)

Foxglove (*Digitalis purpurea*)

Lily of the valley (*Convallaria majalis*)

Kalanchoe (*Bryophyllum* spp.)

Azalea (*Rhododendron* spp.): weakness, hypotension, dyspnea, respiratory failure, GI signs

Yew (*Taxus* spp.): conduction disturbances, bradycardia, GI signs, weakness, seizures; poor prognosis once signs are seen

## Plants Affecting the Gastrointestinal System

Oxalate-containing plants: gastric and ocular irritants

Dumbcane (*Dieffenbachia* spp.)

Philodendron (*Philodendron* spp.)

Peace lily (*Spathiphyllum* spp.)

Devil's ivy (*Epipremnum aureum*)

Rhubarb leaves (*Rheum* spp.)

Philodendron may cause renal and CNS signs in cats.

Chinaberry tree (*Melia azedarach*): vomiting, diarrhea, abdominal pain, hypersalivation; may progress to CNS signs and death

Cycad palms (*Cycas* spp.) or sago palms (*Macrozamia* spp.): vomiting, diarrhea, followed by lethargy, depression, liver failure, and death (dogs)

English ivy (*Hedera helix*): GI irritation, profuse salivation, abdominal pain, vomiting, diarrhea

Castor bean plant (*Ricinus communis*): ricin is among the most deadly poisons in the world; severe abdominal pain, vomiting, diarrhea, seizures, cerebral edema; prognosis for recovery is poor once clinical signs develop.

Holly (*Ilex* spp.), poinsettia (*Euphorbia pulcherrima*), mistletoe (*Phoradendron flavescens*): mild GI irritation, occasionally diarrhea, more serious effects with mistletoe

Amaryllis, jonquil, daffodil (family Amaryllidaceae), tulip (family Liliaceae), iris (family Iridaceae): ingestion of bulb associated with mild-to-moderate gastroenteritis

Autumn crocus *(Colchinum autumnale)*, glory lily *(Gloriosa* spp.): colchicine, vomiting, diarrhea, abdominal pain, hypersalivation progressing to depression, multiple organ system collapse, and death

Solanaceae family: tomato, eggplant, deadly or black night-shade, Jerusalem cherry-solanine, gastric irritant; may cause CNS depression and cardiac arrhythmias; night-shade can also contain belladonna

Mushrooms: amanitin poisoning *(Amanita virosa, Amanita phalloides, Conocybe filaris)*, orellanine poisoning *(Cortinarius orellanus, Cortinarius rainierensis)*, monometh-ylhydrazine *(Gyromitra esculenta)*—severe hepatic disease; survivors of hepatic phase may succumb to renal tubular necrosis

## Plants Affecting the Neurologic System

Tobacco *(Nicotiana tabacum):* vomiting, CNS involvement, cardiac involvement

Hallucinogenic plants: psilocybins or "magic mushrooms," marijuana *(Cannabis sativa)*, jimsonweed *(Datura stramo-nium)*, thorn apple *(Datura metaliodyl)*, blue morning glory *(Ipomoea violacea)*, nutmeg *(Myristica fragrans)*, peyote (family Cactaceae)

Nettle toxicity (family Urticaceae): hunting dogs; toxins contained in needles (histamine, acetylcholine, serotonin, formic acid), salivation, vomiting, pawing at mouth, trem-ors, dyspnea, slow and irregular heartbeat

Macadamia nuts: locomotor disturbances, tremors, ataxia, weakness

Yesterday, today, tomorrow *(Brunfelsia* spp.)

## Plants Affecting the Renal System

Easter lily *(Lilium longiflorum)* and daylily *(Hemerocallis* spp.), possibly other lilies: toxic to cats, vomiting, depression, anorexia, leading to acute renal failure; poor prognosis without early treatment

Raisins/grapes: acute renal failure

## Plants Causing Sudden Death

Seeds of many fruit trees (apple, apricot, cherry, peach, plum), contain cyanogenic glycosides

## Venomous Bites and Stings

### Snakes, Spiders, Others

#### CROTALIDS (PIT VIPERS, RATTLESNAKES, COPPERHEADS, WATER MOCCASINS)

Enzymatic and nonenzymatic proteins, local tissue damage: localized pain, salivation, weakness, fasciculations, hypotension, alterations in respiratory pattern, regional lymphadenopathy, mucosal bleeding, obtundation, convulsions, anemia, echinocytosis, stress leukogram

#### ELAPIDS (CORAL SNAKES)

Rare envenomation, signs delayed 10–18 hours, emesis, salivation, agitation, central depression, quadriplegia, hyporeflexia, intravascular hemolysis, respiratory paralysis

#### *LATRODECTUS* SPP. (WIDOW SPIDERS)

Hyperesthesia, muscle fasciculations, cramping, somatic abdominal pain (characteristic sign), respiratory compromise, hypertension, tachycardia, seizures, agitation, ataxia, cardiopulmonary collapse

#### LOXOSCELIDAE (RECLUSE OR BROWN SPIDERS)

Cutaneous form: bull's-eye lesion, pale center with localized thrombosis, surrounded by erythema, develops into a hemorrhagic bulla with underlying eschar
Viscerocutaneous form: Coombs-negative hemolytic anemia, thrombocytopenia, DIC

#### TICK PARALYSIS

*Dermacentor* and *Haemaphysalis* ticks, ascending paralysis, LMN signs, megaesophagus and aspiration pneumonia in severe cases, spontaneous recovery a few days after tick removal

#### HYMENOPTERAN STINGS

Bites and stings of winged insects and fire ants
Toxic and allergic reactions (localized angioedema, urticaria, emesis, diarrhea, hematochezia, respiratory depression, death)

#### HELODERMATIDAE LIZARD (GILA MONSTER)

Salivation, lacrimation, emesis, tachypnea, respiratory distress, tachycardia, hypotension, shock

# Urogenital Disorders

## Differentiating Between Urine Marking and Inappropriate Elimination in Cats

### Urine Marking

Generally vertical surfaces (can be horizontal)
Marking behavior (may be territorial signaling or an
   anxiety- or conflict-induced response)
Most common in intact males, females in estrus
Adults
Urine (rarely stool)
Doors, windows, new objects, owner's possessions,
   frequently used furniture

### Inappropriate Elimination

Horizontal surfaces (rarely vertical)
Elimination behavior
Males or females, intact or neutered
Any age
Urine and/or stool
Elimination in a variety of areas

## Glomerular Disease

### Types, Dogs and Cats

Immune-complex glomerulonephritis
Membranous glomerulopathy (most common in cats)

Membranoproliferative form
- Type I (mesangiocapillary)
- Type II (dense deposit disease)

Proliferative glomerulonephritis (mesangial and endocapillary)

Crescentic type (rare)

IgA nephropathy

Lupus nephritis

Amyloidosis

Glomerulosclerosis

Focal segmental glomerulosclerosis

Global glomerulosclerosis

Hereditary nephritis

Minimal change glomerulopathy

## Differential Diagnosis for Diseases Associated With Glomerular Disease, Dogs

### INFECTION

*Bacterial*

Pyelonephritis

Pyoderma

Pyometra

Endocarditis

Bartonellosis

Brucellosis

Borreliosis

Anaplasmosis

Other chronic bacterial infections

*Parasitic*

Dirofilariasis

*Heterobilharzia americana*

*Rickettsial*

Ehrlichiosis

*Fungal*

Blastomycosis

Coccidioidomycosis

*Protozoal*

Babesiosis

Hepatozoonosis

Leishmaniasis

Trypanosomiasis

*Viral*

Canine adenovirus (type I) infection

## INFLAMMATION
Periodontal disease
Chronic dermatitis
Pancreatitis
Inflammatory bowel disease
Polyarthritis
SLE
Other immune-mediated diseases

## NEOPLASIA
Lymphosarcoma
Mastocytosis
Leukemia
Systemic histiocytosis
Primary erythrocytosis
Other neoplasms

## MISCELLANEOUS
Corticosteroid excess
Trimethoprim-sulfa therapy
Hyperlipidemia
Chronic insulin infusion
Congenital C3 deficiency
Cyclic hematopoiesis in gray Collies
Masitinib

## FAMILIAL
Amyloidosis (Beagle, English Foxhound)
Hereditary nephritis (Bull Terrier, English Cocker
  Spaniel, Dalmatian, Samoyed)
Glomerulosclerosis (Doberman Pinscher,
  Newfoundland)
Glomerular vasculopathy and necrosis (Greyhound)
Mesangiocapillary glomerulonephritis (Bernese
  Mountain Dog)
Atrophic glomerulopathy (Rottweiler)
Proliferative and sclerosing glomerulonephritis
  (Soft-Coated Wheaten Terrier)

## IDIOPATHIC

# Differential Diagnosis for Diseases Associated With Glomerular Disease, Cats

## INFECTION
### Bacterial
Pyelonephritis
Chronic bacterial infections
Mycoplasmal polyarthritis

*Viral*
>   FIV
>   FIP
>   FeLV

## INFLAMMATION
Pancreatitis
Cholangiohepatitis
Chronic progressive polyarthritis
SLE
Other immune-mediated diseases

## NEOPLASIA
Lymphosarcoma
Leukemia
Mastocytosis
Other neoplasms

## MISCELLANEOUS
Acromegaly
Mercury toxicity

## FAMILIAL

## IDIOPATHIC

## Indications for Cystoscopy

Localization of source of hematuria
Urinary tract neoplasia
- Determine extent and location of tumors
- Obtain samples for cytology or histopathology

Removal of small polyps or tumors
Recurrent urinary tract infections
- Examine for anatomic abnormalities or uroliths
- Obtain samples for cytology, histopathology, or culture

Examine for urachal diverticula
Urinary tract trauma
- Examine for perforations, ruptures, and patency of urinary tract

Urinary incontinence
- Examine for ectopic ureters and/or urethral anomalies
- Laser ablation of intramural ectopic ureters
- Periurethral collagen injections for treatment of refractory urethral incompetence

Urolithiasis
- Confirm and remove small uroliths from bladder or urethra

- Obtain uroliths for quantitative analysis and culture
- Retrieve uroliths from bladder or urethra using stone forceps or stone basket
- Fragment uroliths with laser lithotripsy
- Fill bladder before and after voiding urohydropropulsion to remove small uroliths

## Mammary Masses

### Differential Diagnosis

Benign mammary tumors
- Mixed tumors (fibroadenomas)
- Adenomas
- Mesenchymal tumors

Malignant mammary tumors
- Solid carcinomas
- Tubular adenocarcinomas
- Papillary adenocarcinomas
- Anaplastic carcinomas
- Sarcomas (rare)
- Most feline mammary tumors are adenocarcinomas

Mammary hyperplasia

Mastitis

Granulomas

Duct ectasia

Skin tumors

Lipomas

Foreign bodies (e.g., BB pellets or shot may be confused with small mammary masses)

## Prostatic Disease

### Differential Diagnosis

Benign prostatic hyperplasia (BPH)

Acute prostatitis

Chronic prostatitis

Abscess

Cyst

Prostatic neoplasia
- Adenocarcinoma most common
- Transitional cell carcinoma second most common
- Urothelial carcinoma
- Primary and metastatic hemangiosarcoma
- Lymphoma

## Diagnostic Evaluation

History of lower urinary tract signs, penile discharge, hematuria, dysuria, tenesmus, obstipation, ribbon stools, stiff gait. Severe systemic signs suggest sepsis, or systemic inflammation raises suspicion of acute prostatitis. Intact males are more predisposed to BPH and prostatitis.

Digital rectal examination along with caudal abdominal palpation is a noninvasive initial screening test. The prostate should be bilaterally symmetric, have a smooth and regular surface, have soft parenchyma, and not be painful to touch.

Radiography of limited value for providing an actual diagnosis but may provide information about size, shape, contour, and location of the prostate. Prostatomegaly may cause dorsal displacement of the colon and cranial displacement of the urinary bladder. Mineralization with neoplasia, bacterial prostatitis, and abscessation may be apparent.

Prostatic ultrasound is the most useful and practical imaging method. Normal prostate should have smooth borders and homogenous parenchymal pattern of moderate echogenicity. Ultrasound also offers the opportunity for guided aspirates and core biopsy sampling for culture, cytology, and histopathology.

CT and MRI can evaluate size, shape, and homogeneity of prostate and allow evaluation of intrapelvic lesions, metastatic spread, and ureteral obstruction.

Definitive diagnosis requires cytologic, histologic, or bacteriologic evaluation of a prostate sample. Samples can be obtained using procedures such as semen collection, prostatic massage and wash, brush technique, fine-needle aspiration, and biopsy.

## Proteinuria in Dogs and Cats

### Diagnostic Approach

Stop use of nephrotoxic drugs.

If proteinuria is insignificant (trace to 1+ dipstick reading and urine specific gravity >1.035), there is no need for further workup.

Perform urinalysis to exclude hemorrhage, infection, or inflammation as cause of proteinuria. If these conditions are present, do urine culture. If these conditions are not present, do urine protein/creatinine ratio.

Perform serum chemistry and CBC. Evaluate serum albumin and globulin.

Marked proteinuria ratio (UP/UC >3) with quiet sediment and normal globulins or a polyclonal gammopathy is consistent with renal glomerular disease (glomerulonephritis, amyloidosis). Rule out causes of glomerulonephropathy such as heartworm disease, hepatozoonosis, immune-mediated diseases such as SLE, chronic infectious diseases such as borreliosis, FeLV, FIV, ehrlichiosis, other chronic inflammatory diseases, neoplasia, and hyperadrenocorticism.

If no underlying disease found, may need renal biopsy to assess for glomerulonephritis or amyloidosis

Proteinuria detected by precipitation testing but not dipstick or proteinuria associated with a monoclonal gammopathy may be caused by Bence-Jones proteins. This requires a search for osteolytic or lymphoproliferative lesions. Ehrlichiosis may mimic myeloma. If *Ehrlichia* negative, protein electrophoresis is indicated. A monoclonal gammopathy suggests myeloma.

## Proteinuria Differential Diagnosis

### Prerenal

Physiologic (fever, hyperthermia, seizures, venous congestion, strenuous exercise)

Excessive load (hemoglobinemia, myoglobinemia, severe hyperproteinemia

### Renal

Glomerular
  Glomerulonephritis
    Infectious (chronic bacterial [gingivitis, pyoderma, endocarditis], ehrlichiosis, brucellosis, borreliosis, dirofilariasis, anaplasmosis, leishmaniasis)
    Immune-mediated (SLE, membranoproliferative glomerulonephritis)
    Familial (many breeds, esp. Soft-Coated Wheaten Terrier, Bull Terrier, Dalmatian)
    Neoplastic (lymphoma, mastocytosis, leukemia, histiocytosis)
    Inflammatory (chronic dermatitis, gingivitis, pancreatitis, polyarthritis, inflammatory bowel disease)
    Idiopathic (minimal change disease, membranous nephropathy)

Glomerulosclerosis (systemic hypertension, hyperadre-
nocorticism, diabetes mellitus)
Amyloidosis (inflammatory, familial, idiopathic)
Tubular (Fanconi syndrome, tubular necrosis)

### Post renal

Lower urinary (infectious or sterile cystitis, urolithiasis,
hemorrhagic cystitis, transitional cell carcinoma)
Genital (perivulvar dermatitis, vaginitis, pyometra,
prostatitis)

## Pyelonephritis, Bacterial

### Clinical Findings, Dogs and Cats

Fever
Renal pain
Leukocytosis
Anorexia
Lethargy
Cellular casts in urine sediment
Azotemia
Hematuria
Inability to concentrate urine
Polyuria/polydipsia
Recurrent lower urinary tract infection
Ultrasonographic or excretory urographic abnormalities
• Renal pelvis dilatation
• Asymmetric filling of diverticula
• Dilated ureters
Bacteria in inflammatory lesions on histopathologic
examination
Positive culture of ureteral urine collected by cystoscopy
Positive culture of urine obtained after rinsing bladder with
sterile saline
Positive culture of urine obtained by ultrasound-guided
pyelocentesis

## Renal Disease

(see also Glomerular Disease)

### Familial—Dogs and Cats

Amyloidosis—Beagle, English Foxhound, Shar-Pei,
Abyssinian cat, Oriental shorthaired cat, Siamese cat
Renal Dysplasia—Lhasa Apso, Shih Tzu, Standard Poodle,
Soft-Coated Wheaten Terrier, Chow Chow, Alaskan

Malamute, Miniature Schnauzer, Dutch Kooiker (Dutch decoy dog)

Fanconi syndrome (tubular dysfunction)—Basenji

Tubular dysfunction (renal glucosuria)—Norwegian Elkhound

Basement membrane disorder—Bull Terrier, Doberman Pinscher, English Cocker Spaniel, Samoyed

Membranoproliferative glomerulonephritis—Bernese Mountain Dog, Brittany Spaniel, Soft-Coated Wheaten Terrier

Primary glomerular disease—Rottweiler, Beagle, Pembroke Welsh Corgi, Newfoundland, Bullmastiff, Doberman Pinscher, Dalmatian, Bull Terrier, English Cocker Spaniel, Samoyed

Periglomerular fibrosis—Norwegian Elkhound

Polycystic kidney disease—Cairn Terrier, West Highland White Terrier, Bull Terrier, Persian cat

Multifocal cystadenocarcinoma—German Shepherd

## Differential Diagnosis, Renal Tubular Disease

### CYSTINURIA
Inherited proximal tubular defect
Many breeds of dogs, including mixed breeds
Often leads to cystine calculi formation

### CARNITINURIA
Reported in dogs with cystinuria
May lead to carnitine deficiency and cardiomyopathy

### HYPERURICOSURIA
Abnormal purine metabolism
- Dalmatians
- Dogs with primary hepatic disease
May lead to urate urolithiasis

### HYPERXANTHINURIA (RARE)
Seen in dogs receiving allopurinol to prevent urate uroliths
Congenital hyperxanthinuria seen in a family of Cavalier King Charles Spaniels

### RENAL GLUCOSURIA
Primary renal glycosuria (rare)
- Scottish Terrier, Basenji, Norwegian Elkhound, mixed breeds

### FANCONI SYNDROME
Inherited proximal tubular defect
Basenjis most common
May lead to renal failure

## RENAL TUBULAR ACIDOSIS

Rare tubular disorders that lead to hyperchloremic metabolic acidosis
- Proximal renal tubular acidosis
- Distal renal tubular acidosis

## NEPHROGENIC DIABETES INSIPIDUS

Any renal disorder that suppresses the kidneys' response to ADH

Congenital (rare)

Acquired
- Toxic (*Escherichia coli* endotoxin)
- Drugs (glucocorticoids, chemotherapeutics)
- Metabolic disease (hypokalemia, hypercalcemia)
- Tubular injury or loss (polycystic renal disease, bacterial pyelonephritis)
- Medullary washout

## Differentiating Acute From Chronic Renal Failure

### ACUTE RENAL FAILURE

History of ischemia
History of exposure to toxin
Active urine sediment
Good body condition
Hyperkalemia (if oliguric)
Normal-to-increased hematocrit
Enlarged kidneys
Potentially severe metabolic acidosis
Severe clinical signs for level of dysfunction
Normal-sized parathyroid glands (ultrasound appearance)
Not polyuric/polydipsic

### CHRONIC RENAL FAILURE

History of previous renal disease
History of polyuria/polydipsia
Small irregular kidneys
Nonregenerative anemia
Normal to hypokalemia
Normal-to-mild metabolic acidosis
Inactive urine sediment
Weight loss/cachexia
Mild clinical signs for level of dysfunction
Enlarged parathyroid glands (ultrasound appearance)

# Renal Toxins in Dogs and Cats

## THERAPEUTIC AGENTS

### *Antibacterial Agents*
Aminoglycosides
Sulfonamides
Nafcillin
Penicillins
Cephalosporins
Fluoroquinolones
Carbapenems
Rifampin
Tetracyclines
Vancomycin

### *Antifungal Agents*
Amphotericin B

### *Antiviral Agents*
Acyclovir
Foscarnet

### *Antiprotozoal Agents*
Pentamidine
Sulfadiazine
Trimethoprim-sulfamethoxazole
Dapsone

### *Anthelmintics*
Thiacetarsamide

### *Cancer Chemotherapeutics*
Cisplatin/carboplatin
Methotrexate
Doxorubicin
Azathioprine

### *Immunosuppressive Drugs*
Cyclosporine
Interleukin-2

### *NSAIDs*

### *ACE Inhibitors*

### *Diuretics*

### *Miscellaneous Agents*
Dextran 40
Allopurinol
Cimetidine
Apomorphine
Deferoxamine

Streptokinase
Methoxyflurane
Penicillamine
Acetaminophen
Tricyclic antidepressants

*Radiocontrast Agents*

## NONTHERAPEUTIC AGENTS

*Heavy Metals*
Lead
Mercury
Cadmium
Chromium

## ORGANIC COMPOUNDS

Ethylene glycol
Carbon tetrachloride
Chloroform
Pesticides
Herbicides
Solvents

## MISCELLANEOUS AGENTS

Mushrooms
Snake venom
Grapes/raisins
Bee venom
Lily

*Pigments*
Hemoglobin/myoglobin

*Hypercalcemia*

## Causes of Acute Renal Failure in Dogs and Cats

### PRIMARY RENAL DISEASE

*Infection*
Pyelonephritis
Leptospirosis
Infectious canine hepatitis
Borreliosis
FIP

*Immune-Mediated Disease*
Acute glomerulonephritis
SLE
Renal transplant rejection

*Renal Neoplasia*
Lymphoma

## NEPHROTOXICITY
Exogenous toxins
Endogenous toxins
Drugs

## RENAL ISCHEMIA
*Prerenal Azotemia*
Dehydration/hypovolemia
Deep anesthesia
Sepsis
Shock/vasodilation
Decreased oncotic pressure
Hyperthermia
Hypothermia
Hemorrhage
Burns
Transfusion reaction

*Renal Vascular Disease*
Avulsion
Thrombosis
Stenosis

## SYSTEMIC DISEASES WITH RENAL MANIFESTATIONS
Infection
- Bacterial endocarditis
- FIP
- Borreliosis
- Babesiosis
- Leishmaniasis

Pancreatitis
Diabetes mellitus
Hyperadrenocorticism
Hypoadrenocorticism
Hypocalcemia
Hypokalemia
Hypomagnesemia
Hyponatremia
SIRS
Sepsis
Multiple organ failure
DIC
Heart failure
SLE
Hepatorenal syndrome
Malignant hypertension
Hyperviscosity syndrome
- Polycythemia

* Multiple myeloma

Urinary outflow obstruction

Envenomation

## Causes of Chronic Renal Failure in Dogs and Cats

Inflammatory/infectious
* Pyelonephritis
* Leptospirosis
* Blastomycosis
* Leishmaniasis
* FIP

Familial/congenital (see p. 296)

Amyloidosis

Neoplasia
* Lymphosarcoma
* Renal cell carcinoma
* Nephroblastoma
* Tumor lysis syndrome
* Others

Nephrotoxicants (see p. 299)

Renal ischemia

Sequela of acute renal failure

Glomerulopathies (see p. 291)

Nephrolithiasis

Bilateral hydronephrosis
* Spay granulomas
* Transitional cell carcinoma at trigone obstructing both ureters
* Nephrolithiasis

Polycystic kidney disease

Urinary outflow obstruction

Idiopathic

## Penis, Prepuce, and Testes Disorders—Differential Diagnosis

### ACQUIRED PENILE DISORDERS

Penile trauma
* Hematoma
* Laceration
* Fracture of os penis

Priapism (abnormal, persistent erection)

Neoplasia

Vesicles

Warts

Ulcers

Penile urethral obstruction
Penile urethral prolapse

## CONGENITAL PENILE DISORDERS

Persistent penile frenulum
Penile hypoplasia
Hypospadias (defect in closure of urethra)
Diphallia (duplication of penis)

## PREPUTIAL DISORDERS

Balanoposthitis
- Bacterial infection
- Blastomycosis
- Canine herpesvirus

Phimosis
Paraphimosis

## TESTICULAR DISORDERS

Cryptorchidism
Orchitis/epididymitis
- *Mycoplasma* spp.
- *Brucella canis*
- *Blastomyces* spp.
- *Ehrlichia* spp.
- Rocky Mountain spotted fever
- FIP

Testicular torsion
Scrotal dermatitis
Testicular neoplasia
- Sertoli cell tumor
- Leydig cell tumor
- Seminoma

## DRUGS AND METABOLIC DISORDERS AFFECTING MALE REPRODUCTION

Glucocorticoids (hyperadrenocorticism, exogenous glucocorticoids)
Decreased luteinizing hormone (LH), testosterone, sperm output, seminal volume, and libido; increased sperm abnormalities
Estrogens, androgens, anabolic steroids
Decreased LH, testosterone, and spermatogenesis
Cimetidine
Decreased testosterone, libido, and sperm count
Spironolactone, anticholinergics, propranolol, digoxin, verapamil, thiazide diuretics, chlorpromazine, barbiturates, diazepam, phenytoin, primidone
Decreased testosterone and libido
Progestogens, ketoconazole

Decreased testosterone
Amphotericin B, many anticancer drugs
Decreased spermatogenesis
Diabetes mellitus
Decreased libido and sperm count, abnormal semen
Renal failure, stress
Decreased libido and sperm count

## Ureteral Diseases

### Differential Diagnosis

#### VESICOURETERAL REFLUX
Primary: 7–12 weeks old—intrinsic maldevelopment of ureterovesical junction, self-limiting
Secondary to lower urinary tract obstruction, UTI, surgical damage, neurologic disease of bladder, ectopic ureters

#### CONGENITAL ANOMALIES
Ectopic ureters
Ureterocele
Ureter agenesis
Ureter duplication
Urethrorectal or urethrovaginal fistula

#### ACQUIRED URETERAL DISEASE
Ureteral trauma
- Blunt trauma
- Penetrating trauma
- Iatrogenic damage during surgery

Inadvertent ligation and transection during ovariohysterectomy
Urinoma (paraureteral pseudocyst)
Ureteral obstruction
- Intraluminal (blood clot, calculus)
- Intramural (fibrosis, stricture, neoplasia)
- Extramural (retroperitoneal mass, bladder neoplasia, inadvertent ligature)

Calculi (nephroliths or nephrolith fragments that have migrated into the ureter)
- Calcium oxalate (most common in cat)
- Struvite (both struvite and calcium oxalate are most common in dog)

Neoplasia
- Transitional cell carcinoma
- Leiomyoma
- Leiomyosarcoma

- Sarcoma
- MCT
- Fibroepithelial polyp
- Benign papilloma
- Metastatic neoplasia

## Urinary Tract Infection

## Clinical Findings

### LOWER URINARY TRACT INFECTION

Dysuria

Pollakiuria

Urge incontinence/inappropriate urination

Gross hematuria at end of micturition

Cloudy urine

Foul odor to urine

Small, painful, thickened bladder

Palpable urocystoliths

Asymptomatic

Pyuria

Hematuria

Proteinuria

Bacteriuria

Normal CBC

Perivulvar dermatitis

### UPPER URINARY TRACT INFECTION

Polyuria/polydipsia

Signs of systemic illness or infection

Possible renal failure

Fever

Abdominal pain

Kidneys normal to enlarged

Leukocytosis

Pyuria

Hematuria

Proteinuria

Bacteriuria

Cellular or granular casts

Decreased urine specific gravity

Recurrent lower UTI

### ACUTE PROSTATITIS OR PROSTATIC ABSCESS

Urethral discharge independent of micturition

Signs of systemic illness/infection

Dysuria, hematuria, pollakiuria, pyuria, urinary
   incontinence

Fever
Painful prostate or abdomen
Tenesmus
Prostatomegaly/asymmetry
Leukocytosis ($\pm$)
Pyuria
Hematuria
Proteinuria
Bacteriuria
Inflammatory prostatic cytology

### CHRONIC PROSTATITIS
Recurrent UTIs
Urethral discharge independent of urination
Possible dysuria
Normal CBC
Pyuria
Hematuria
Proteinuria
Bacteriuria
Prostatomegaly/asymmetry

## Canine Lower Urinary Tract Disease—Differential Diagnosis

### UROCYSTOLITHS
Struvite (magnesium ammonium phosphate)
Calcium oxalate
Purine (urate/xanthine)
Cystine
Calcium phosphate
Silica
Compound uroliths

### URETHRAL OBSTRUCTION
Urethroliths (see Urocystoliths)
Blood clots
Urethral stricture
Neoplasia
- Transitional cell carcinoma
- Prostatic adenocarcinoma
- Leiomyoma
- Leiomyosarcoma
- Prostatic adenocarcinoma
- Squamous cell carcinoma
- Myxosarcoma
- Lymphoma
- MCT

Proliferative urethritis
Urinary bladder entrapment in perineal hernia
Trauma
- Penile fracture

### URINARY TRACT TRAUMA
Contusion (bladder or urethra)
Urethral tears
Rupture of bladder (blunt trauma, secondary to pelvic fracture, penetrating wound)
Avulsion of bladder or urethra
Penile fracture

### INFLAMMATION (BLADDER OR URETHRA)
Bacterial UTI
Fungal UTI
Polypoid cystitis
Emphysematous cystitis
Cyclophosphamide-induced cystitis
Parasitic cystitis (*Capillaria plica*)

## Feline Lower Urinary Tract Disease—Differential Diagnosis

Feline idiopathic cystitis
Urethral plug (obstructive feline idiopathic cystitis)
Urolithiasis
- Struvite
- Calcium oxalate
- Urate
- Cystine

Bacterial cystitis (less common in cats than in dogs)
Stricture
Neoplasia

## Uroliths, Canine

### Characteristics

#### CALCIUM OXALATE MONOHYDRATE OR DIHYDRATE
Radiopaque
Acidic to neutral pH
Sharp projections or smooth uroliths; calcium oxalate dihydrate uroliths may be jackstone shaped
Not associated with urinary tract infection
Calcium oxalate dihydrate crystals: square envelope shape
Calcium oxalate monohydrate crystals: dumbbell shaped

### STRUVITE (MAGNESIUM AMMONIUM PHOSPHATE)
Radiopaque
Alkaline pH
Smooth to speculated if single; smooth and pyramidal in shape if multiple
Associated with infection with urease-producing bacteria (*Staphylococcus, Proteus, Ureaplasma* spp., *Klebsiella, Corynebacterium*)
"Coffin lid"–shaped crystals

### URATE/XANTHINE
Radiolucent to faintly radiopaque
Acidic pH
Smooth uroliths
Not associated with infection
Yellow-brown "thorn apple" (spherical) or amorphous crystals

### CYSTINE
Faintly to moderately radiopaque
Acidic pH
Smooth, round uroliths; staghorn-shaped uroliths if nephroliths present
Not associated with infection
Hexagonal-shaped crystals

### CALCIUM PHOSPHATE
Radiopaque
Alkaline to normal pH for hydroxyapatite, acidic for brushite
Small, variably shaped uroliths for hydroxyapatite
Smooth, round or pyramidal for brushite
Not associated with infection
Amorphous phosphate crystals or thin prisms (calcium phosphate)

### SILICA
Radiopaque
Acidic to neutral pH
Jackstone-shaped uroliths
Not associated with infection
No crystals

## Vaginal Discharge

## Differential Diagnosis

### CORNIFIED EPITHELIAL CELLS
Normal proestrus
Normal estrus

Contamination of skin or epithelium
Ovarian remnant syndrome
Abnormal source of estrogen
- Exogenous
- Ovarian follicular cyst
- Ovarian neoplasia
Contamination of squamous epithelium

## MUCUS
Normal late diestrus or late pregnancy
Normal lochia
Mucometra
Androgenic stimulation

## NEUTROPHILS
### Nonseptic (No Microorganisms Seen)
Vaginitis
Normal first day of diestrus
Metritis or pyometra

### Septic
Vaginitis
Metritis
Pyometra
Abortion

## PERIPHERAL BLOOD
Subinvolution of placental sites
Uterine or vaginal neoplasia
Trauma to reproductive tract
Uterine torsion
Coagulopathies

## CELLULAR DEBRIS
Normal lochia
Abortion

# Pain Diagnosis

Acute Pain Assessment
Acute Pain Preemptive Scoring System (Examples in Each Category)
Chronic Pain Assessment

## Acute Pain Assessment

Subjective evaluation of pain in animals relies on observation and interpretation of animal behavior. Pain may be indicated by loss of normal behaviors or appearance of abnormal behaviors.

### Dogs

Restless, agitated, delirious, circling, thrashing
Lethargic, withdrawn, dull, obtunded
May ignore environmental stimuli
Abnormal sleep–wake cycle, inability to sleep
May bite, lick, or chew painful area
Adopt abnormal body positions to cope with pain, hunched posture, "prayer position"
Abnormal tail position
Lameness, abnormal gait
Anorexia, reluctant to eliminate
Ears held back, eyes wide open with dilated pupils or closed with a dull appearance
Disuse or guarding of painful area
Vocalization (whimper, yelp, whine, groan, yowl)
May become more aggressive and resist handling or palpation, or may become more timid and seek increased contact with caregivers

### Cats

Hide, stay to back of cage
Behavior may be mistaken for fear or anxiety
May sit very quietly, and pain may be missed by those looking for more active signs of pain
May continue to purr while in pain
May growl with ears flattened
May attempt escape
Lack of grooming
Hunched posture, statuelike appearance
Reduced or absent appetite
Tail flicking

## Acute Pain Preemptive Scoring System (Examples in Each Category)

### Minor Procedures: No Pain

Physical examination, restraint
Radiography
Suture removal, cast application, bandage change
Grooming
Nail trim

### Minor Surgeries: Minor Pain

Suturing, debridement
Urinary catheterization
Dental cleaning
Ear examination and cleaning
Abscess lancing
Removing cutaneous foreign bodies

### Moderate Surgeries: Moderate Pain

Ovariohysterectomy, castration, cesarean section
Feline onychectomy
Cystotomy
Anal sacculectomy
Dental extraction
Cutaneous mass removal
Severe laceration repair
Eye surgery, enucleation

### Major Surgeries: Severe Pain

Fracture repair, cruciate ligament repair
Thoracotomy, laminectomy, exploratory laparotomy
Limb amputation
Ear canal ablation

## Chronic Pain Assessment

Clinical signs of chronic pain depend on underlying cause and pathologic state.
Range from subtle to obvious
May see acute flareups that require changes in treatment (e.g., osteoarthritic dog that experiences acute pain after excessive strenuous activity)
Decreased activity
Reluctance to rise or play
Changes in sleep patterns

Changes in appetite
Changes in social interaction and grooming habits
Withdrawal, aggression
Owner observations are extremely important.

# FAST Ultrasound

FAST Ultrasound Examinations (Focused Assessment With Sonography for Trauma, Triage, and Tracking)

TFAST as an Extension of the Physical Exam

## FAST Ultrasound Examinations (Focused Assessment With Sonography for Trauma, Triage, and Tracking)

### GFAST (Global FAST) is the Combination of AFAST, TFAST, and Vet BLUE

GFAST should be used as an extension of the physical exam in sick or injured patient. With training, all three FAST exams can be completed in about 5 minutes.

### AFAST (Abdominal FAST)

#### PROCEDURE

Patients are placed in either lateral recumbency; right is preferred because the basic echo views, gallbladder, caudal vena cava, left kidney are more easily imaged. Dorsal recumbency should not be used because of increased patient respiratory and hemodynamic stress.

Ultrasound probe is placed in four regions of abdomen:

- Diaphragmatic–hepatic (DH) view—at the level of the xiphoid, images the diaphragm, liver, gallbladder, caudal vena cava, pleural space, pericardial space, and lung
- Spleno renal (SR) view—images spleen, left kidney, abdominal and retroperitoneal spaces
- Cysto colic (CC) view—images bladder; however, an air-filled colon can confound imaging
- Hepato renal (HR) Umbilical view—images small intestine and spleen
- Probe is fanned in longitudinal (sagittal); transverse is not necessary
- Purpose is quick assessment of AFAST target organs and detection of free abdominal and retroperitoneal fluid. Blood rapidly defibrinates in blunt trauma and nontrauma, so it is seen as anechoic black triangulations. Penetrating trauma is different initially because blood often clots and blends in as soft tissue.

## Abdominal Fluid Score

Four-point scale where 0 means scanned negative for fluid at all four views and 4 means fluid detected at all 4 views

## Application of Abdominal Fluid Score in Medical vs. Surgical Decisions in Bleeding Dogs

### BLUNT TRAUMA (THINK MEDICAL FIRST)

Abdominal fluid score (AFS) 1 and 2 are major injury, small-volume bleeder—no blood transfusion needed, not expected to be anemic (polycythemia vera [PCV] >35%) if intraabdominal bleeding only. Reassess by AFAST and AFS to monitor for changes minimally 4 hours post admission and sooner if unstable. If AFS stays 1–2, but PCV drops, look for bleeding at another site (retroperitoneal, pleural space, fracture site, external).

AFS 3 and 4 are major injury, large-volume bleeder (AFS 3–4 or becomes AFS 3–4). Expect anemia (PCV <35%), use graduated fluid therapy (one-third shock dose), and repeat titrated fluid challenge as needed. With severe anemia (PCV <25%), blood transfusion is often necessary and surgery uncommon.

### PENETRATING TRAUMA (THINK SURGERY WITH ANY POSITIVE AFS)

Blood from ripping, tearing, crushing tends to clot, making it blend with adjacent tissue and difficult to detect by AFAST. With time, clotted blood will defibrinate and become visible as black anechoic triangulations. Serial exams are key and should be performed as often as needed until certain the patient is medical and not surgical.

Combine with other clinical findings such as hernia, refractory pain, septic abdomen, free air to decide between surgical vs. medical.

### POSTINTERVENTIONAL BLEEDING—POSTSURGICAL, POSTPERCUTANEOUS BIOPSY/ASPIRATE, LAPAROSCOPY, INTERVENTIONAL RADIOLOGY, BLEEDING TUMOR, ETC. (THINK MEDICAL FOR AFS 1–2, SURGICAL FOR AFS 3–4)

AFS 3 and 4 initially or on serial exams need surgical ligation of bleeding.

AFS 1 and 2 that stays 1 or 2 with serial exams is not surgical.

AFS 3 and 4 that are not anemic still need surgical exploration; waiting may lead to need for transfusion and additional risk and expense.

Nontraumatic hemoabdomen (variably medical and
surgical)

- Bleeding intraabdominal tumor, spleen most common,
  PCV generally low normal or low. Surgical problem.
- Canine anaphylaxis, PCV generally high normal or
  above normal. Look for gallbladder wall edema called
  *striation* or *halo sign*. Medical problem.
- Coagulopathy is an uncommon cause of nontraumatic hemoabdomen. Correct coagulopathy if present. Medical problem.

## AFAST as an Extension of the Physical Exam

### DIAPHRAGMATIC–HEPATIC VIEW

DH and CC views are most common positive sites in
low-scoring dogs and cats.

Useful for detecting pericardial effusion (racetrack sign)
and pleural effusion

Advantage: less air interference than transthoracic
TFAST views

Assessment of the weak or collapsed patient's volume
status by observing dynamics of caudal vena cava
(CVC) as it passes through diaphragm

- A distended caudal vena cava with little variability in
  its diameter supports a high central venous pressure
  (CVP) and hypervolemia; CVC is fat often accompa-
  nied by hepatic venous distension (tree trunk sign).
  Rule-outs include:
- Right-sided volume overload
- Pulmonary hypertension
- Right-sided heart failure
- Dilated cardiomyopathy
- An attenuated CVC with little variability in its diam-
  eter supports a low CVP and hypovolemia; CVC is flat.
- Rule-outs include causes of profound hypovole-
  mia, including hypovolemia and distributive shock
  (anaphylaxis, hemorrhage, gastric dilatation-volvulus
  [GDV], sepsis).
- The CVC normally has a change in its diameter of
  between 30% and 50%, in the ballpark of normal
  with a "bouncing" appearance.
- Gallbladder is often adjacent the diaphragm on DH
  view.
- May be displaced by an enlarged liver
- May be difficult to image with diaphragmatic hernia
  or gallbladder rupture, calculi/mineralization, or
  emphysema

- Feline gallbladders are more difficult to image on DH view
- Gallbladder wall edema, intramural sonographic striation, has been referred to as the "halo" *sign*
- May be indicative of canine anaphylaxis in acute collapse/weakness
- May be indicative of right-sided heart failure, pericardial effusion/tamponade in acute collapse/weakness
- May be indicative of volume overload, third spacing, primary gallbladder disease, and pancreatitis in the less acute patient
- Liver masses, cysts, and diffuse or irregular changes in echogenicity may be appreciated

## SPLENORENAL VIEW

Least gravity-dependent view where air would rise to (pneumoabdomen) and fluid only at this site may be retroperitoneal rather than intraabdominal

Acoustic window into the abdominal and retroperitoneal space for free abdominal fluid and retroperitoneal fluid

Splenic masses and diffuse or irregular changes in echogenicity may be appreciated.

Left kidney may appreciate variety of pathology, including hydronephrosis, pyelectasia, cortical cysts, perinephric cysts, masses, mineralization, calculi, and mineralization.

May be able to also see right kidney in small dogs and cats through the SR view

## CYSTOCOLIC VIEW

CC and DH views are most common positive site in low-scoring dogs and cats.

Urinary bladder may appreciate variety of lesions such as calculi, masses, wall thickening/abnormalities, and emphysema.

Bladder length (cm) × width (cm) × height (cm) × 0.625=estimated bladder volume in (ml)

## HEPATORENAL UMBILICAL VIEW

Spleen and small intestine most often visible here.

Splenic masses and diffuse or irregular changes in echogenicity may be appreciated.

Small intestine pathology may be appreciated, including dilated loops (ileus, obstruction), wall thickening, masses, and related lymph nodes.

The name of this view is a misnomer because the liver and right kidney are not typically imaged.

Liver and right kidney are normally not present at the
level of the umbilicus unless they are enlarged.

Stomach is not visible at the level of the umbilicus
unless it is distended.

The HR umbilical view completes AFAST and is likely the
region to perform abdominocentesis in higher-scoring
dogs and cats.

## TFAST (Thoracic FAST)

### PROCEDURE

Patients may be positioned in right or left lateral recumbency, especially if TFAST examination pericardial site
(PCS) views immediately follow the AFAST examination in stable patients, and in respiratory-compromised
patients, and for the chest tube site (CTS) view; sternal
recumbency or standing positioning is safer and preferred for the entire TFAST examination.

Ultrasound probe is placed in five positions:

- DH view—immediately caudal to the xiphoid (same
  as AFAST DH view). Useful for detecting pericardial
  effusion (racetrack sign) and pleural effusion.
- Left and right CTS views—at the level of the seventh
  to eighth intercostal spaces at the highest point,
  upper third of the thorax, where lung may be visualized on the dorsolateral thoracic wall in the absence
  of pneumothorax, and where the cap of air would rise
  in the presence of pneumothorax

If evidence of lung against the thoracic wall is observed
sonographically, then pneumothorax is effectively
ruled out.

If there is no evidence that lung is against the thoracic
wall, then the lung point is searched for where the
transition zone is between pneumothorax and lung
recontacting the thoracic wall.

- Left and right PCS view—over the heart at the level
  of the fifth and sixth intercostal spaces in gravity-
  dependent regions of the thorax

PCS views are used for quick assessment of lungs, heart,
pleural, and pericardial spaces.

## TFAST as an Extension of the Physical Exam

### Diaphragmatic–Hepatic View

Part of both AFAST and TFAST examinations—see AFAST
Diaphragmatic–Hepatic View

Useful for sonographic confirmation of pleural effusion and pericardial effusion (racetrack sign)

Less air interference than TFAST transthoracic PCS views, liver and gallbladder provide acoustic window into thorax

Allows for assessment of volume status by observing dynamics of the CVC (see Diaphragmatic–Hepatic View in AFAST as an Extension of Exam).

## Chest Tube Site View

Useful for ruling out pneumothorax and for surveying for lung lesions

Probe is placed perpendicular to the long axis of the adjacent ribs in order to image the intercostal space.

The orientation obtained is referred to as the gator (alligator) *sign* from the image created by rounded rib heads as the gator's eyes, and the intercostal space, a white line, as the bridge of the gator's nose, likened to a partially submerged alligator peering at the sonographer.

Glide sign—normal to-and-fro motion of lung along the intercostal space or more specifically, the movement of parietal and visceral pleura, ruling out pneumothorax; absence of the glide sign suggests pneumothorax.

B-lines (also called ultrasound lung rockets, ULRs)—hyperechoic streaks that extend from pleural line through the far field that oscillate like a pendulum in synchrony with respiration

- Trauma-associated B-lines immediately rule out pneumothorax at that level of the thorax and support lung contusions until proven otherwise.
- In nontrauma, B-lines represent various forms of alveolar-interstitial edema, including left-sided CHF, hemorrhage, variety of pneumonias, inflammation, as more common causes (see Vet BLUE).

Step sign—deviation from the expected linear pulmonary–pleural interface

- Chest wall trauma or disease (intercostal tears, fractured ribs, subpleural hematoma)
- Pleural space disease (effusion, diaphragmatic hernia, masses)

Lung point—location or transition zone at which collapsed lung secondary to pneumothorax recontacts thoracic wall

- Move probe ventrally to middle, then ventral or lower third of the thorax with patient standing or sternal until evidence of lung against the thoracic wall is found, then move incrementally dorsally until lung is lost to determine the exact lung point

- Use the lung point to assess and monitor pneumothorax; upper one-third is trivial to mild; middle one-third is moderate; lower one-third is severe

## Pericardial Site Views

Used to visualize the heart, pericardial space, and pleural space

Assess for pericardial or pleural effusion combining with the DH view

Increase depth so that the heart is seen in its entirety to avoid false-positives from mistaking right ventricle/other heart chambers for effusion

TFAST echo views: left ventricular short axis view to assess volume status and contractility; long axis four-chamber view to assess for right-sided conditions; short axis LA:Ao ratio (left atrium:aorta) for left-sided conditions

## Clinical Indications and Applications of TFAST

Blunt trauma
Penetrating trauma
Undifferentiated hypotension
Collapse/apparent collapse
Acute cardiopulmonary decompensation
Pulmonary contusion
Detection of atrial tears
Postinterventional (thoracic surgery, lung lobe aspirate, thoracoscopy, tracheal wash, thoracentesis, chest tube)
Monitoring pneumothorax
Pleural and pericardial effusion
Detecting and monitoring forms of pulmonary edema and respiratory distress
Patient monitoring during fluid resuscitation

## Vet BLUE Lung Ultrasound

### PROCEDURE

Probe is positioned as described at the TFAST CTS view but then moved through three more views bilaterally

Vet BLUE has eight total acoustic views (four views bilaterally)

- Caudodorsal lung region (Cd)—same as TFAST CTS view, upper third of the thorax at the level of the eighth to ninth intercostal spaces directly above the xiphoid, near the highest point where lung may be visualized on the dorsolateral thoracic wall
- Perihilar lung region (Ph)—sixth to seventh intercostal space, middle third of the thorax

- Middle lung region (Md)—fourth to fifth intercostal space, lower third of the thorax
- Cranial lung region (Cr)—second to third intercostal space, lower third of the thorax

The most recent, most accurate described methodology by the originator of the Vet BLUE is to begin by finding the transition zone in a standing (or sternal) patient at the CTS/Cd view where abdominal contents and lung are viewed over an intercostal space, then sliding toward the head two intercostal spaces to begin the Vet BLUE at the Cd view (point 1).

From the Cd view (point 1), draw an imaginary line to the elbow. Halfway from the Cd to the elbow is the Ph view (point 2), and at the elbow is the Md view (point 3), and then in the axillary area as the final Cr view. If the heart is in view at the Md, slide the probe directly dorsally until over lung for the Md view, and define the Cr view by finding the transition of lung and thoracic inlet, then slide caudally over the first two intercostal spaces. If a gator sign orientation is not observed, then you cannot be assured the lung is being imaged.

## Vet BLUE Lung Ultrasound Findings in Progression From Most to Least Aerated/ Most Consolidated

Dry lung—glide sign with A-lines (reverberation artifact) at lung line indicates dry lung at the lung periphery. The confounder: A-lines with no glide sign consistent with pneumothorax.

Wet lung B-lines (also called ULRs)—hyperechoic streaks that oscillate with respiration and extend to the far field, obliterating A-lines.

Shred sign—deviation of the lung line (pulmonary–pleural line) and within the deviation, hyperechoic foci of air movement seen in bronchi. Comparable to a radiographic air bronchogram. Indicates lung consolidation/infiltration.

Tissue sign—more severe consolidation/infiltration where no air movement is present. Referred to as hepatization of lung.

Nodule sign—anechoic round (nodule), often with a hyperechoic far border and acoustic enhancement through the far field as a B-lines.

## Vet BLUE Differential Diagnosis for Patients With Respiratory Signs With Dry Lung in All Fields

### RESPIRATORY

Upper airway disease (laryngeal paralysis, collapsing trachea)

Airway obstruction (mass)

Feline asthma

Chronic obstructive pulmonary disease

Pulmonary thromboembolism

Centrally located lung lesion away from lung line, therefore missed by Vet BLUE

### CARDIAC

Cardiac arrhythmia

Dilated cardiomyopathy

Cardiac tamponade

### UNDIFFERENTIATED HYPOTENSION

Canine anaphylaxis

Cavitary hemorrhage (hemoabdomen, hemothorax, hemoretroperitoneum)

Sepsis

### OTHER NONRESPIRATORY

High fever

Heat stroke

Severe metabolic acidosis

Severe anemia

## GFAST Triad for Volume Status and Patient Monitoring

GFAST, the name for the use of AFAST and its fluid scoring system, TFAST and Vet BLUE combined, may be used for rapid patient volume status assessment during, before, and after fluid resuscitation.

- Characterization of CVC and hepatic veins for estimation of CVP (see AFAST as an Extension of the Physical Exam, Diaphragmatic-Hepatic View); forms of shock (e.g., hypovolemic/distributive shock/cardiogenic/obstructive shock)
- TFAST—assessment of cardiac views for volume and contractility, right- and left-sided conditions (see TFAST)
- Vet BLUE—presence of wet lung screens for left-sided cardiac overload, and the pattern-based approach and Vet BLUE lung ultrasound signs help determine CHF, pneumonia, neoplasia, granulomatous conditions, pulmonary thromboembolism ( PTE), and others

# PART THREE

# LABORATORY VALUES AND
# INTERPRETATION OF RESULTS

*Note: Normal ranges are meant to provide the reader with an approximation of normal. Individual laboratory values should be compared with the reference range values of the laboratory that performed the test.*

## Acetylcholine Receptor Antibody

***Normal Range***
Feline: <0.3 nmol/L
Canine: <0.6 nmol/L

***Elevated in:*** myasthenia gravis

*Note: A positive titer is diagnostic for myasthenia gravis. Negative titers occur in 10%–20% of positive cases; therefore, a negative titer does not exclude myasthenia gravis.*

## Activated Coagulation Time (ACT)

***Normal Range***
Feline: <165 seconds
Canine: 60–110 seconds
   Screening test for intrinsic and common coagulation pathways (factors II, V, VIII, IX, X, XI, XII); may also be prolonged with severe thrombocytopenia and decreased fibrinogen

## Activated Partial Thromboplastin Time (aPTT)

***Normal Range***
Feline: 10–19 seconds
Canine: 9–17 seconds
Determines abnormalities in the intrinsic coagulation
    pathway
Prolonged with deficiencies in factors VIII, IX, XI, and XII and
    fibrinogen; also prolonged with disseminated intravascular
    coagulation (DIC)
Prolonged with von Willebrand disease, acquired vitamin K
    deficiency, coumarin poisoning, bile insufficiency, liver
    failure
Severely prolonged with hemophilia A (factor VIII deficiency)
    and hemophilia B (factor IX)

## Adrenocorticotropic Hormone (ACTH), Endogenous

*Normal Range*
Feline: not reported
Canine: 10–70 pg/mL

*Elevated in:*
pituitary-dependent hyperadrenocorticism, hypocortisolemia in primary hypoadrenocorticism

*Decreased in:*
iatrogenic Cushing syndrome and adrenal tumors

## Adrenocorticotropic Hormone (ACTH) Stimulation Test

*Normal Range*
*Pre-ACTH injection*
Feline: 1.0–4.5 μg/dL
Canine: 2–6 μg/dL

*Post-ACTH injection*
Feline: 4.5–15.0 μg/dL (13–16 μg/dL: suggestive of hyperadrenocorticism, >16 μg/dL strongly suggestive)
Canine: 5.5–20.0 μg/dL (18–24 μg/dL: suggestive of hyperadrenocorticism, >24 μg/dL strongly suggestive)
From 15%–20% are false-negative results; false-positive results may be seen with stress or nonadrenal illness
Pre-ACTH cortisol is in normal range, and post-ACTH cortisol shows little to no change with iatrogenic Cushing syndrome
Pre-ACTH cortisol is below normal, and post-ACTH cortisol shows little change with hypoadrenocorticism
Pre-ACTH and post-ACTH cortisol levels should be between 1 and 5 μg/dL with successful mitotane induction or while on maintenance Lysodren therapy
Trilostane induction: <1.45 μg/dL, stop treatment; restart on a lower dose
1.45–5.4 μg/dL, continue on same dose
5.4–9.1 μg/dL, continue on current dose if clinical signs well controlled or increase dose if clinical signs of hyperadrenocorticism still evident
>9.1 μg/dL, increase initial dose

*Note: ACTH stimulation does not differentiate pituitary-dependent hyperadrenocorticism from adrenal tumors. The low-dose dexamethasone test is more diagnostic for canine Cushing syndrome.*

## Alanine Aminotransferase (ALT, Formerly SGPT)

*Normal Range*
Feline: 10–100 IU/L
Canine: 12–118 IU/L

*Elevated in:*
hepatocellular membrane damage and leakage
*Inflammation:* chronic active hepatitis, lymphocytic/plasma-
cytic hepatitis (cats), enteritis, pancreatitis, peritonitis,
cholangitis, cholangiohepatitis
*Infection:* bacterial hepatitis, leptospirosis, feline infectious
peritonitis (FIP), infectious canine hepatitis
*Toxicity:* chemical, heavy metals, mycotoxins
*Neoplasia:* primary, metastatic
*Drugs*
*Endocrine:* diabetes mellitus, hyperadrenocorticism,
hyperthyroidism
*Trauma*
*Hypoxia:* cardiopulmonary disease, thromboembolic disease
*Metabolism:* feline hepatic lipidosis, storage diseases (e.g., copper)
*Liver lobe torsion*
*Hepatocellular regeneration*
*Cirrhosis*

*Decreased in:*
end-stage liver disease, but in most cases, decreased ALT is not
significant

## Albumin

*Normal Range*
Feline: 2.5–3.9 g/dL
Canine: 2.7–4.4 g/dL

*Elevated in:*
dehydration (globulin and total protein should also be
increased), spurious (e.g., hemolysis, lipemia, laboratory error),
higher in adults than in juveniles

*Decreased in:*
protein-losing nephropathy (amyloidosis, glomerulonephritis,
glomerulosclerosis), gastroenteropathy (malabsorption, maldigestion, protein-losing enteropathy), liver failure, portosystemic shunt, malnutrition (dietary, parasitism), exudative skin
disease (vasculitis, burns, abrasions, degloving injury), neonates,
external blood loss, compensatory (chronic effusions, hyperglobulinemia, multiple myeloma)

## Aldosterone

*Normal Range*
Feline: resting or pre-ACTH 194-388 pmol/L, post 277-721 pmol/L
Canine: resting or pre-ACTH 14-957 pmol/L, post 197-2103

*Elevated in* Adrenal neoplasia, low sodium uptake, nonadrenal disease that result in hypovolemia or hyponatremia

*Decreased in*
hypoadrenocorticism, adrenal atrophy (idiopathic, secondary to medication, pituitary disease, high sodium intake)

## Alkaline Phosphatase, Serum (SAP or ALP)

*Normal Range*
Feline: 6–102 IU/L
Canine: 5–131 IU/L

*Elevated in:*
biliary tract abnormalities (pancreatitis, bile duct neoplasia, cholelithiasis, cholecystitis, ruptured gallbladder); hepatic parenchymal disease (cholangitis/cholangiohepatitis, chronic hepatitis, nodular hypoplasia, copper storage disease, hepatic lipidosis [cats], cirrhosis, hepatic neoplasia [lymphoma, hemangiosarcoma, hepatocellular carcinoma, metastatic carcinoma], toxic hepatitis, FIP [cats]); corticosteroids; anticonvulsants (phenobarbital, primidone); endocrine disorders (diabetes mellitus, hyperadrenocorticism [dogs], hyperthyroidism [cats]); enteritis; bone isoenzyme (fracture repair, osteosarcoma); young dog with bone growth; osteosarcoma; osteomyelitis; ehrlichiosis; diaphragmatic hernia; passive congestion due to right heart failure; iatrogenic

Note: Almost any disorder that affects the liver can cause elevations in SAP levels.

## Ammonia

*Normal Range*
Feline: 30–100 µg/dL
Canine: 45–120 µg/dL

*Elevated in:*
hepatic failure (portosystemic shunt, cirrhosis); postprandial, postexercise (racing dogs), spurious (e.g., hemolysis, lipemia, laboratory error)

*Note: Due to instability of samples, this test has mostly been replaced by serum bile acids.*

## Amylase, Serum

*Normal Range*
Feline: 100–1200 U/L
Canine: 290–1125 U/L

*Elevated in:*
pancreatitis, pancreatic neoplasia, pancreatic duct obstruction, pancreatic necrosis, enteritis, renal disease (decreased filtration of amylase)

*Note: Serum amylase levels may not correlate with severity of disease. Not very sensitive or specific, especially in cats*

## Anion Gap

*Normal Range*
Feline: 12–24 mEq/L
Canine: 16.3–28.6 mEq/L

### Laboratory Calculation

$$[Na + K] - \left[ Cl + HCO_3^- \right] = \text{Anion gap}$$

*Elevated in:*
metabolic acidosis from acids that do not contain chloride (lactic acidosis, uremia, ketoacidosis, ethylene glycol toxicosis). Metabolic acidosis with normal anion gap has an increased plasma chloride concentration and is called hyperchloremic acidosis.

*Decreased in:*
hypoalbuminemia, IgG multiple myeloma

## Antinuclear Antibody (ANA)

*Normal Range*
Reported as a titer, very laboratory dependent. Refer to your
    laboratory for normal ranges
High positive titer, with associated clinical and clinico-
    pathologic signs, supports a diagnosis of systemic lupus

erythematosus (SLE). Many immune-mediated, inflammatory, and infectious diseases and neoplasms can result in low positive titers. Results may be false-negative with chronic glucocorticoid use

## Antithrombin (AT)

*Normal Range*
Measured as a percentage of species-specific pooled samples
Dogs: 75%–120%
Cats: 75%–110%

*Elevated in:*
exogenous glucocorticoid administration (dogs); inflammation; elevation of antithrombin is not clinically significant

*Decreased in:*
decreased production (hepatopathy, portosystemic shunt); increased loss (protein-losing nephropathy, glomerulonephritis, renal amyloidosis, protein-losing enteropathy); increased hepatic clearance of antithrombin enzyme complexes (DIC, sepsis)

Often decreased in patients with DIC, nephrotic syndrome, and thrombosis; AT levels of <70% of the control cause the patient to be unresponsive to heparin therapy without first providing AT replacement therapy

## Arterial Blood Gases

*Normal Range*

|  | Canine | Feline |
|---|---|---|
| pH | 7.35–7.45 | 7.36–7.44 |
| $PaCO_2$ | 36–44 | 28–32 |
| $PaO_2$ | 90–100 | 90–100 |
| $TCO_2$ | 25–27 | 21–23 |
| $HCO_3^-$ | 24–26 | 20–22 |

## Blood Gas Interpretation

### EVALUATE $PAO_2$

*Hypoxemia*

Arterial oxygen tension/partial pressure ($PaO_2$) of less than 85 mm Hg

Emergency treatment for hypoxemia needed when $PaO_2$ is less than 60 mm Hg

Cyanosis may be seen when $PaO_2$ is 50 mm Hg or lower, depending on hemoglobin concentration.

*Potential Causes of Hypoxemia*

Right-left shunts (patent ductus arteriosus, ventricular septal defects, intrapulmonary shunts)

Ventilation/perfusion mismatch (various pulmonary diseases)

Diffusion impairment

Hypoventilation (anesthesia, neuromuscular disease, airway obstruction, central nervous system disease, pleural space or chest wall abnormality)

Decrease in fraction of inspired oxygen (hooked up to empty oxygen tank)

### Evaluate pH:

increase in pH: alkalemia (metabolic alkalosis or respiratory alkalosis)

decrease in pH: acidemia (metabolic acidosis or respiratory acidosis)

### Assess Acid–Base Status:

*If acidemic:*

Arterial carbon dioxide tension ($PaCO_2$) elevated: respiratory acidosis

$PaCO_2$ decreased: compensatory respiratory alkalosis

Bicarbonate ($HCO_3^-$) decreased: metabolic acidosis

$HCO_3^-$ elevated: compensatory metabolic alkalosis

*If alkalotic:*

$PaCO_2$ decreased: respiratory alkalosis

$PaCO_2$ elevated: compensatory respiratory acidosis

$HCO_3^-$ elevated: metabolic alkalosis

$HCO_3^-$ decreased: compensatory metabolic acidosis

## Aspartate Aminotransferase (AST, Formerly SGOT)

Not considered clinically significant in the dog or cat

Very sensitive but not very specific; significant amounts of AST found also in muscle

## Bartonella

Bacteria of the genus *Bartonella* infect at very low levels, so even a highly sensitive polymerase chain reaction (PCR) assay may not detect bacterial DNA in the patient sample. Traditional testing methodologies such as immunofluorescence antibody (IFA) or Western blot analysis are therefore likely to produce false-negative results.

Preenrichment cultures of samples with *Bartonella alpha* Proteobacteria Growth Media (BAPGM) followed by PCR greatly improves sensitivity, and this methodology has become the gold standard for diagnosis. This combination of test methods increases the likelihood of detecting *Bartonella* infection by supporting the growth of any viable bacterium up to levels detectable by DNA amplification.

## Recommendations for Testing

Tissue and nonblood fluid samples: Preliminary testing results indicate that *Bartonella*-positive results from preenrichment and PCR are obtained more often from tissue and nonblood fluid samples than from blood. Accordingly, it is recommended to test specimens drawn from as close as possible to the area of disease pathology.

Triple draws: *Bartonella* cycles in a relapsing pattern of bacteremia. The odds of detecting a positive *Bartonella* infection are increased significantly by blood draws on 3 separate days over the course of a week, refrigerated, and submitted all at once for testing.

Serology testing: Although preenrichment and PCR testing significantly increase the odds of detecting active *Bartonella* infection, serologic testing for antibodies also provides important diagnostic support to confirm exposure and to potentially implicate infection that may have been missed by DNA testing. The best patient care information is obtained by combining results of serology and the preenrichment and PCR.

Posttreatment followup: *Bartonella* infections can be difficult to clear with either single or combination antibiotics. Followup testing is recommended 4–6 weeks after treatment or at regular intervals posttreatment depending on patient status.

Preenrichment and PCR testing and serologic testing are all available at GALAXY Diagnostics, www.galaxydx.com.

## Basophil Count

### Normal Range
Feline: 0–150 cells/µL
Canine: 0–150 cells/µL

### Elevated (basophilia) in:
Disorders associated with IgE production/binding (heartworm disease, atopy, flea allergy), allergic reactions (e.g., food, insect sting), inflammatory disease (gastrointestinal [GI] tract disease, respiratory tract disease), neoplasia (mast cell neoplasia,

basophilic leukemia, lymphomatoid granulomatosis), myelo-proliferative diseases (essential thrombocythemia, polycythemia vera), associated with hyperlipoproteinemia and possibly hypothyroidism

## Bence-Jones Proteinuria

Excessive immunoglobulin light chains in the urine
A positive result is abnormal in the dog and the cat.

### Elevated in
lymphoproliferative disease (multiple myeloma, lymphoma)
Chronic infectious diseases (e.g. ehrlichiosis, babesiosis, leishmaniasis)

## Bicarbonate (HCO$_3^-$)

### Normal Range
Feline: 20–22 mmol/L
Canine: 24–26 mmol/L

*If acidemic:*

### Elevated in:
metabolic alkalosis (with compensatory acidosis)

### Decreased in:
metabolic acidosis

*If alkalotic:*

### Elevated in:
metabolic alkalosis

### Decreased in:
metabolic acidosis (with compensatory alkalosis)

## Bile Acids

### Normal Range
Preprandial: Feline and canine: 0–5.0 μmol/L
Postprandial:
Feline: 1–20.0 μmol/L
Canine: 5.0–25.0 μmol/L

### Elevated in:
hepatocellular disease, cholestatic disease, portosystemic shunt, biliary rupture

### Decreased in:
Delayed gastric emptying, malabsorption disorders, rapid intestinal transport, ileal resection

Patient must be fasted and cannot be icteric. Typically measure preprandial and 2-hour postprandial serum samples

May also measure urine bile acids, although patients with portosystemic shunts tend to have lower urine bile acids than patients with hepatocellular disease

## Bilirubin

### Normal Range
Feline: <1.0 mg/dL
Canine: <1.0 mg/dL

### Elevated in:
prehepatic, hemolysis (intravascular or extravascular), cholestasis (extrahepatic [pancreatitis, cholangitis, cholecystitis, cholelithiasis, biliary neoplasia], intrahepatic [nodular hyperplasia, feline hepatic lipidosis, cholangitis/cholangiohepatitis, cirrhosis, hepatic lymphoma, acute hepatic necrosis]), duodenal perforation, ruptured gallbladder

## Blood Urea Nitrogen (BUN)

### Normal Range
Feline: 14–36 mg/dL
Canine: 6–25 mg/dL

### Elevated in:
prerenal azotemia (dehydration, hypoadrenocorticism, heart failure, shock, GI hemorrhage, high-protein diet); increased catabolism (fever, drugs, [e.g., tetracycline]); renal failure; pyelonephritis; postrenal azotemia (urethral [obstruction, urolith, urethral tear, plant awn]; bladder [obstruction, urolith, blood clot, polyp, neoplasia, rupture])

### Decreased in:
diuresis (polydipsia, hyperadrenocorticism, overzealous fluid therapy, drugs [e.g., glucocorticoids], diabetes insipidus [DI]); liver failure (portosystemic shunt, cirrhosis, urea cycle enzyme deficiency); low-protein diet; malnutrition; neonates

## Buccal Mucosal Bleeding Time (BMBT)

*Normal Range*
Feline and canine: <3 minutes
Prolonged bleeding time is a sensitive and specific indicator of diminished platelet function (e.g., severe thrombocytopenia, von Willebrand disease, and uremia)

## Calcium (Ca)

*Normal Range*
Feline: 8.2–10.8 mg/dL
Canine: 8.9–11.4 mg/dL

*Elevated in:*
primary hyperparathyroidism; renal failure; hypoadrenocorticism; hypercalcemia of malignancy (lymphosarcoma, apocrine gland adenocarcinoma, carcinomas [nasal, mammary gland, gastric, thyroid, pancreatic, prostate, pulmonary]; osteolytic [multiple myeloma, lymphosarcoma, squamous cell carcinoma, osteosarcoma, fibrosarcoma]); hypervitaminosis D (cholecalciferol rodenticides, plants, excessive supplementation); dehydration; granulomatous disease (systemic mycosis [blastomycosis], schistosomiasis, FIP); nonmalignant skeletal disorder (osteomyelitis, hypertrophic osteodystrophy [HOD]); iatrogenic disorder (excessive calcium supplementation, excessive oral phosphate binders); factitious disorders (serum lipemia, postprandial measurement, young animal); laboratory error; idiopathic (cats)

*Decreased in:*
renal failure (acute and chronic); acute pancreatitis; intestinal malabsorption; primary hypoparathyroidism (idiopathic, postthyroidectomy); puerperal tetany (eclampsia); ethylene glycol toxicity; hypoproteinemia/hypoalbuminemia; hypomagnesemia; nutritional secondary hyperparathyroidism; tumor lysis syndrome; phosphate-containing enemas; anticonvulsant medications; hypovitaminosis D, rhabdomyolysis, sodium bicarbonate administration; laboratory error

## Cerebrospinal Fluid (CSF)

*Normal Range*
Normal CSF is colorless and clear. Discoloration usually means red blood cells (RBCs) or neutrophils are present.

| Value | Canine | Feline | Cytology (%) | | |
|---|---|---|---|---|---|
| WBCs ($\times 10^3$/L) | $\leq 3$ | $\leq 2$ | Monocytes | 87 | 69–100 |
| RBCs ($\times 10^6$/L) | $\leq 30$ | $\leq 30$ | Lymphocytes | 4 | 0–27 |
| Protein (mg/dL) | $\leq 33$ | $\leq 36$ | Neutrophils | 3 | 0–9 |
| | | | Eosinophils | 0 | 0 |
| | | | Macrophages | 6 | 0–3 |

*Infectious central nervous system (CNS) disease:* increased white blood cells (WBCs) and protein content

*Inflammatory CNS disease:* increased WBCs and protein content

*Brain neoplasia:* normal to mild elevation of WBCs, mild elevation of protein content

*Hydrocephalus, lissencephaly:* normal WBCs and protein content

*Degenerative myelopathy, intervertebral disk disease, polyradiculoneuritis:* normal WBCs and normal to mildly increased protein content

Most common cause of RBCs in CSF is contamination during collection

## Chloride (Cl)

### Normal Range
Feline: 104–128 mEq/L
Canine: 102–120 mEq/L
Often changes proportionally with sodium; in those cases, it is usually easier to search for the cause of the sodium change

#### CORRECTED HYPERCHLOREMIA (ELEVATION OF CHLORIDE DISPROPORTIONATE TO ELEVATION OF SODIUM)

*Excessive Loss of Sodium Relative to Chloride*
Small bowel diarrhea (common and important)

*Pseudohyperchloremia*
Lipemic samples using colorimetric methods
Potassium chloride therapy (common and important)

*Excessive Gain of Chloride Relative to Sodium*
Therapy with chloride salts ($NH_4Cl$, KCl)
Total parenteral nutrition
Fluid therapy (0.9% NaCl, hypertonic saline, KCl-supplemented fluids)
Salt poisoning
Renal chloride retention (renal failure, renal tubular acidosis, hypoadrenocorticism, diabetes mellitus,

chronic respiratory alkalosis, drug-induced [acetazolamide, spironolactone])

Exercise (endurance exercise in sled dogs; short, submaximal exercise [agility])

## CORRECTED HYPOCHLOREMIA (LOSS OF CHLORIDE RELATIVE TO SODIUM)

### Gastrointestinal Loss

Vomiting of stomach contents

Selected GI diseases associated with hyperkalemia and hyponatremia in dogs without hypoadrenocorticism (trichuriasia, salmonellosis, perforated duodenal ulcer)

### Renal Loss

Therapy with thiazide or loop diuretics

Chronic respiratory acidosis

Hyperadrenocorticism

Glucocorticoid administration

### Therapy With Solutions With High Sodium Concentration Relative to Chloride

Sodium bicarbonate

Exercise in racing Greyhounds

## Cholesterol (CH)

*Normal Range*
Feline: 75–220 mg/dL
Canine: 92–324 mg/dL

*Elevated in:*
postprandial, primary hyperlipidemia, endocrine disorders (hypothyroidism, hyperadrenocorticism, diabetes mellitus), cholestasis, dietary (high-cholesterol diet), nephrotic syndrome, protein-losing nephropathy, idiopathic (Doberman Pinscher, Rottweiler)

*Decreased in:*
liver failure, malabsorption, maldigestion, protein-losing enteropathy, portosystemic shunt, lymphangiectasia, starvation, hypoadrenocorticism, selected malignancies

## Cholinesterase

*Normal Range*
Feline: 500–4000 U/L
Canine: 800–4000 U/L

***Decreased in***
organophosphate toxicity, carbamate toxicity

## Cobalamin

***Normal Range***
Feline: 290–1499 pg/mL
Canine: 251–908 pg/mL

***Decreased in:***
exocrine pancreatic insufficiency, distal small intestinal disease, diffuse small intestinal disease, small intestinal bacterial overgrowth (usually combined with an increased serum folate level), hepatic disease in cats

## Complete Blood Count (CBC)

***Normal Range***

### TOTAL WHITE BLOOD CELL COUNT
Feline: 3.5–16.0×103/μL
Canine: 4.0–15.5×10³/μL

### TOTAL RED BLOOD CELL COUNT
Feline: 5.92–9.93×106/μL
Canine: 4.8–9.3×10⁶/μL

### HEMOGLOBIN
Feline: 9.3–15.9 g/dL
Canine: 12.1–20.3 g/dL

### HEMATOCRIT (PACKED CELL VOLUME [PCV])
Feline: 29%–48%
Canine: 36%–60%

### RETICULOCYTE COUNT
Feline: 0%–10.5% punctate or 0%–1.0% aggregate
Canine: 0%–1.0% aggregate

### MEAN CORPUSCULAR VOLUME (MCV)
Feline: 37–61 fL
Canine: 58–79 fL

### MEAN CORPUSCULAR HEMOGLOBIN (MCH)
Feline: 11–21 pg
Canine: 19–28 pg

### MEAN CORPUSCULAR HEMOGLOBIN CONCENTRATION (MCHC)
Feline: 30–38 g/dL
Canine: 30–38 g/dL

**PLATELET COUNT**
Feline: 200–500 103/μL
Canine: 170–400 $10^3$/μL

**TOTAL SOLIDS**
Feline: 5.2–8.8 g/dL
Canine: 5.0–7.4 g/dL

## Coombs Test

Indicates presence of antibody and/or complement on the surface of erythrocytes; supports the diagnosis of immune-mediated hemolytic anemia

## Cortisol

*Normal Range*
Feline and canine: 1.0–4.5 μg/dL
Not a reliable indicator of disease; considerable overlap between normal patients and those with adrenal disease

*Elevated in:*
stress (environmental, illness), drugs (prednisone and predniso-lone [may cross-react in assay], anticonvulsants), pituitary- and adrenal-dependent hyperadrenocorticism

*Decreased in:*
Drugs (steroids, trilostane, mitotane, ketoconazole) [suppression of adrenal function]), hypoadrenocorticism

## Creatine Kinase (CK, Formerly CPK)

*Normal Range*
Feline: 56–529 U/L
Canine: 59–895 U/L

*Elevated in:*
trauma, myositis (immune-mediated, eosinophilic myositis, masticatory muscle myositis, infectious [toxoplasmosis, neo-sporosis], endocarditis), exertional myositis, surgery (tissue damage), nutritional (hypokalemia [polymyopathy], taurine deficiency), prolonged recumbency, intramuscular injections, pyrexia, hypothermia, postinfarct ischemia (cardiomyopathy, DIC), muscle ischemia secondary to status epilepticus

## Creatinine

*Normal Range*
Feline: 0.6–2.4 mg/dL
Canine: 0.5–1.6 mg/dL

*Elevated in:*
azotemia (prerenal, renal, postrenal, rhabdomyolysis)

*Decreased in:*
any condition that causes decreased muscle mass, increased glomerular filtration rate

## Cytologic Criteria of Malignancy

### General Criteria

Anisocytosis and macrocytosis—variation in cell size
Hypercellularity—increased cell exfoliation due to decreased cell adherence
Pleomorphism—variable size and shape of cells of the same type

### Nuclear Criteria

Macrokaryosis—increased nuclear size; nuclei larger than 20 μ suggestive of neoplasia
Increased nucleus-to-cytoplasm ratio (N:C)—normal non-lymphoid cells have usually have a N:C of 1.3:1.8. Ratios of 1.2 or less suggestive of malignancy
Anisokaryosis—variation in nuclear size; especially important if the nuclei of multinucleated cells vary in size
Multinucleation—especially important if the nuclei vary in size
Increased mitotic figures—mitosis is rare in normal tissues
Abnormal mitosis—improper alignment of chromosomes
Coarse chromatin pattern—may appear ropy or cordlike
Nuclear molding—deformation of nuclei by other nuclei within the same cell or adjacent cells
Macronucleoli—nucleoli are increased in size (>5 μ suggestive of malignancy, for reference, RBCs are 5–6 μ in the cat and 7–8 μ in the dog)
Angular nucleoli—fusiform or have other angular shapes instead of their normal round to slightly oval shape
Anisonucleoliosis—variation in nucleolar shape or size (especially important if the variation is within the same nucleus)

## Cytologic Features of Discrete Cell (Round Cell) Tumors

### Discrete Cells (Round Cells)

Present individually in tissues, not adhered to other cells for connective tissue matrix

Most discrete cells are of hematogenous origin.

Aspirates of normal lymphoid tissues like spleen and lymph nodes yield discrete cells.

Discrete cell patterns in other tissues indicate the presence of a discrete cell tumor (round cell tumor).

Cells tend to be small-to-medium sized and round.

### Specific Discrete Cell Tumors

#### MAST CELL TUMOR

Highly cellular smears of predominately mast cells

- Small, red-purple intracytoplasmic granules
- Number of granules seen vary from few to so many the cytoplasm is packed with granules; some mast cells may degranulate during aspiration; more granules in background, fewer in cells.
- Anaplastic mast cell tumors may be virtually devoid of granules.

#### LYMPHOMA

Most cases of lymphoma in dogs and cats are high-grade tumors composed mostly of large blastic lymphoid cells. Cytology typically shows greater than 50% of cells are large, blastic lymphocytes. Lymphoblasts have a high N:C ratio and intensely basophilic cytoplasm.

- Low-grade, well-differentiated lymphoma may yield predominately small lymphocytes. Such tumors are difficult to differentiate from normal or reactive lymphoid tissue and require biopsy and histopathology/immunohistochemistry.

#### CANINE CUTANEOUS HISTIOCYTOMA

Benign tumors of dendritic cell origin, common in young dogs.

- Medium-sized cells, round to oval nuclei that may be indented. Finely stippled chromatin with indistinct nucleoli. Moderate amount of light blue-gray cytoplasm.
- Most histiocytomas regress spontaneously. The presence of small lymphocytes with these tumor cells may be seen in tumors that are regressing.

## MALIGNANT HISTIOCYTOSIS/HISTIOCYTIC SARCOMA/ SYSTEMIC HISTIOCYTOSIS

Cytologic appearance varies from benign-looking cells to populations of histiocytic cells with marked atypia.

- Common features include large discrete cells with abundant vacuolated cytoplasm, prominent cytophagia, and multinucleation. May demonstrate marked anisocytosis, anisokaryosis, and variation of N:C ratio. Macrocytosis, karyomegaly, and large multinucleated cells are common.
- Definitive diagnosis may not be possible based on cytology alone.

## PLASMACYTOMA

Tumors of plasma cell origin include multiple myeloma (arising primarily from bone marrow) and extramedullary plasmacytomas (usually cutaneous but may be in other sites, such as GI).

- Cutaneous plasmacytomas are usually benign. GI tumors are more likely to be malignant.
- Well-differentiated plasmacytomas yield cells that resemble normal plasma cells. Small, round nuclei with deeply basophilic cytoplasm exist with or without the characteristic paranuclear clear zone. Poorly differentiated plasmacytoma cells are less distinct and demonstrate significant criteria of malignancy. Binucleate and multinucleate cells are common in both well- and poorly differentiated plasmacytomas. This and a lack of lymphoglandular bodies help differentiate these tumors from lymphosarcoma.

## TRANSMISSIBLE VENEREAL TUMOR (TVT)

TVT cells are typically more pleomorphic than other discrete cell tumors.

- Moderate smoky to light blue cytoplasm, numerous cytoplasmic vacuoles that may also be found extracellularly. Nuclei show moderate to marked anisokaryosis and have coarse nuclear chromatin. Nucleoli may be prominent, and mitotic figures are common.

## MELANOMA

Great imitators, cells show features of discrete cells, epithelial cells, or mesenchymal cells. Usually easily recognized due to their pigment. Individual melanin granules are rod-shaped and stain dark green to black. Cells may be heavily to sparsely pigmented.

- Poorly differentiated melanomas may have sparse pigmentation and show marked criteria of malignancy.

## Cytologic Features of Mesenchymal Cells

Mesenchymal cells are cells that form connective tissue, blood vessels, and lymphatics.

Hematopoietic cells are classified as mesenchymal cells, but because their appearance is so distinct, they are typically considered a separate classification. Usually, discussion of mesenchymal cells implies stromal connective tissue cells.

Cytoplasmic borders are often indistinct.

Most connective tissues exfoliate no cells when sampled by fine-needle aspiration. May see fibroblasts or fibrocytes on occasion. Reactive fibroblasts may be seen in aspirates of inflamed tissue or tissues undergoing tissue repair. Reactive fibroblasts may show many criteria of malignancy, but reactive fibroblasts should be suspected when seen within a population of inflammatory cells.

Highly cellular smears that contain predominately a pure population of mesenchymal cells are likely to indicate a mesenchymal neoplasm (sarcoma).

Mesenchymal cells are often elongated with cytoplasm that tapers in one or more directions (referred to as *spindle cells*).

May see elongated cells with rod-shaped nuclei to plump, minimally tapered cells with round nuclei. Neoplastic mesenchymal cell tumors may show features more consistent with epithelial or discrete cells.

## Cytologic Features of Normal Epithelial Cells

Cell-to-cell adhesion

Although normal epithelial cells can be small to large, they can be very large and have abundant cytoplasm.

Round to columnar to caudate in shape and have sharply defined cytoplasmic borders

Nuclei generally are round to oval.

Squamous epithelial cells tend to be more individually oriented when collected by surface swabs or scrapings. As they mature, their nuclei become small and pyknotic, and eventually the cell becomes anucleate.

Respiratory and GI cells are distinctly columnar. May show long rows of cells with nuclei lined up at the basal end. Cilia may be seen at the apical end of respiratory epithelial cells.

Glandular epithelial cells may show evidence of tubular or acinar formation.

Tumors of epithelial cell origin may retain characteristic features.

## Cytology of Ear Canal Swabs

### Bacteria

Ear canals normally contain small amounts of bacteria.

With bacterial otitis, large numbers of bacteria are seen free in the smear.

Neutrophilic inflammation is sometimes seen, especially with concurrent otitis media.

Visualization of cocci on the smear often represents *Staphylococcus* but may also be *Enterococcus* or *Streptococcus*.

Rods most commonly indicate *Pseudomonas*, followed by *Proteus* and *Escherichia coli*.

### Fungi

*Malassezia pachydermatis* is by far the most common yeast seen on ear cytologies but may be found in smaller numbers in normal ears.

May see concurrent bacteria and yeast infection

Yeasts overgrow when the environment is favorable.

Rarely see *Candida* and *Microsporum*

### Mites

*Otodectes cynotis* common primary cause of otitis (50% of cats, 5% of dogs).

*Demodex canis* and *D. cati, Sarcoptes scabiei*, and *Notoedres cati* are infrequently seen in ear canals.

Mites tend to wash off slides during staining. Unstained slides of ear secretions or swabs rolled in mineral oil may be better for finding mites in the ear canal. Skin scrapings of the ear pinna are best for finding *Demodex, Sarcoptes*, or *Notoedres*.

### Neoplasia

The most common benign tumors seen in the ear canal are polyps, papillomas, basal cell tumors, and ceruminous gland adenomas.

The most common malignant tumors are ceruminous gland adenocarcinomas, squamous cell carcinomas, and other carcinomas.

Unfortunately, neoplastic cells are rarely seen on ear cytologies.

May only see cytologic evidence of inflammation

Fine-needle aspiration or biopsy of otic masses is usually necessary to establish a diagnosis.

## Miscellaneous

Ceruminous otitis externa is associated with seborrheic conditions.

Oily, yellow discharge may resemble purulent exudate, but cytology is relatively devoid of inflammatory cells.

## Cytology of Nasal Swabs or Flush Specimens

### Normal Findings

*Simonsiella* spp.—large, stacked, rod-shaped bacteria, normal inhabitants of the oral cavity

Nonkeratinized squamous epithelial cells, often with adherent bacteria, are obtained from the external nares and oropharynx.

Ciliated pseudostratified columnar epithelial cells and mucus from nasal turbinates

Basal epithelial cells are smaller and rounded and have dark blue cytoplasm.

May see RBCs from hemorrhage secondary to sampling.

### Infectious Agents

Neutrophils predominate with bacterial, viral, or fungal infections.

May also see macrophages, lymphocytes, and plasma cells

Bacterial infection suspected when bacteria seen within neutrophils

Because bacteria from the oral cavity are usually a pleomorphic population, monomorphic populations suggest infection.

Bacterial infection of the nasal cavity usually is secondary to trauma, foreign bodies, viral or fungal infection, neoplasia, or oronasal fistulas.

Intranuclear viral inclusions may be seen in epithelial nuclei with herpes infections in cats.

Fungal hyphae may be present; may need special stains to identify. Nasal cavity fungi include *Aspergillus* spp., *Penicillium* spp., *Cryptococcus neoformans, Rhinosporidium* spp.

Nasal mites *(Pneumonyssus caninum, Linguatula serrata).*

*Capillaria aerophila* may be found in nasal sinuses.

### Noninfectious Conditions

Foreign bodies often consist of inhaled plant material (grass awns or foxtails).

May lead to chronic rhinitis

Exudates with eosinophils may be seen with inhaled allergens.

Neoplasia of the nasal cavity is usually seen in older
patients.

Epithelial, mesenchymal tumors of nasal cavity cells, extension of oral neoplasms, or transplanted from other sites
(e.g., TVT).

Most nasal tumors are epithelial in origin.
Adenocarcinomas most common, followed by squamous
cell carcinomas and undifferentiated carcinomas.

Mesenchymal tumors of the nasal cavity include fibrosar-
comas, chondrosarcomas, osteosarcomas, hemangiosarcomas, and undifferentiated sarcomas. Do not exfoliate
readily.

Round cell tumors of the nasal cavity include transmissible
venereal tumors, lymphosarcomas, and mast cell tumors.

## Dexamethasone Suppression Tests

### Low-Dose Dexamethasone Suppression Test (LDDST)

***NORMAL***

Four-hour cortisol level suppresses to less than 50% of baseline
cortisol (usually <1.4 µg/dL), and then 8-hour cortisol
remains at or near that level.

#### PITUITARY-DEPENDENT HYPERADRENOCORTICISM (PDH)

Four-hour cortisol level is suppressed to less than 50% of
baseline (60% of dogs) or <1.4 µg/dL (25% of dogs), and
an 8-hour cortisol level of <50% of baseline but 1.4 µg/
dL or greater (25% of dogs).

Dexamethasone resistance, in which none of the
previous criteria are met, occurs in 40% of PDH cases.

#### FUNCTIONAL ADRENAL TUMOR (FAT)

Dexamethasone administration has no effect on cortisol
levels.

### High-Dose Dexamethasone Suppression Test

Differentiates PDH from FAT in cases where none of the
criteria for PDH is met with the LDDST.

#### FUNCTIONAL ADRENAL TUMOR

Eight-hour cortisol level—no suppression of cortisol
levels with dexamethasone administration

#### PITUITARY-DEPENDENT HYPERADRENOCORTICISM

Eight-hour cortisol level is less than 50% of baseline
cortisol or less than 1.4 µg/dL.

## Disseminated Intravascular Coagulation, Diagnostic Tests

### FIBRINOGEN
increased

### ACTIVATED PARTIAL THROMBOPLASTIN TIME (APTT)
prolonged

### PROTHROMBIN TIME (PT)
prolonged

### PLATELET COUNT
decreased

### FIBRIN DEGRADATION PRODUCTS (ASSAYS FOR BREAKDOWN OF FIBRIN CLOTS)
increased

### D-DIMER (ASSAYS FOR PROTEOLYTIC FRAGMENT OF FIBRINOGEN DEGRADATION)
increased

*Note: D-dimer has a high negative predictive value. A negative test reliably rules out DIC.*

*D-dimer elevation can be seen without hypercoagulability (internal hemorrhage, hepatic disease, renal disease) so it is only recommended when DIC or thrombosis is suspected.*

## Eosinophil Count

*Normal Range*
Feline: 0–1000 cells/μL
Canine: 0–1200 cells/μL

## Eosinophils

*Elevated (eosinophilia) in*
parasitic disorders (hookworm, dirofilariasis, dipetalonemiasis, fleas, filaroides, aelurostrongylus, roundworms, paragonimiasis, *Cuterebra*); hypersensitivity (flea allergy dermatitis, atopy, food allergy); eosinophilic infiltrative disease (eosinophilic granuloma complex, feline bronchial asthma, eosinophilic gastroenteritis/colitis, pulmonary infiltrates with eosinophils [dogs], hypereosinophilic syndrome); infectious diseases (toxoplasmosis, suppurative processes); neoplasia (eosinophilic leukemia, mast cell neoplasia, lymphoma, myeloproliferative disorders, solid tumors), hypoadrenocorticism, pregnancy

*Decreased (eosinopenia) in*
stress, hyperadrenocorticism, glucocorticoid therapy

## Erythrocyte Count (RBC Count)

*Normal Range*
Feline: 5.92–9.93 106/µL
Canine: 4.8–9.3 $10^6$/µL

*Elevated in*
dehydration, splenic contraction, polycythemia (high altitude, left-to-right cardiac shunts, chronic pulmonary disease, paraneoplastic production of erythropoietin rarely seen with renal tumors, polycythemia)

*Decreased in*
regenerative anemias
- Acute and chronic hemorrhage
  - GI hemorrhage
    - Ulcer disease
    - Neoplasia
- Trauma
- Coagulopathies
- Ectoparasites (fleas, ticks)
- Endoparasites (hookworms, *Coccidia*)
- Hematuria

Hemolytic anemia
- Immune-mediated
- Cold hemagglutinin disease
- Oxidant injury (onion, kale, phenothiazines, methylene blue)
- Parasitic
  - Babesiosis
  - *Haemobartonella felis (Mycoplasma haemofelis)*
  - *Haemobartonella canis (Mycoplasma haemocanis)*
  - *Cytauxzoon felis*
  - Infectious
    - Leptospirosis
    - *E. coli*
  - Microangiopathic
    - Dirofilariasis
    - Vascular neoplasia
    - Vasculitis
    - DIC
- Zinc or copper toxicosis
- Hypophosphatemia
- Pyruvate kinase deficiency
- Phosphofructokinase deficiency

Nonregenerative anemias
- Renal failure

- Anemia of chronic disease
  - Inflammatory disease
  - Infectious disease
  - Neoplasia
- Drugs
  - Chemotherapeutics
  - Chloramphenicol
  - Sulfadiazine
  - Phenylbutazone
- Iron deficiency
  - Chronic blood loss
  - Nutritional
- Endocrine disease
  - Hypothyroidism
  - Hypoadrenocorticism
  - Hyperestrogenism
    - Diethylstilbestrol
    - Estradiol
    - Sertoli cell tumor
- Infectious
  - Feline leukemia virus (FeLV)
  - Feline immunodeficiency virus (FIV)
  - Ehrlichiosis
  - Feline panleukopenia virus

Idiopathic aplastic anemia
Red cell aplasia
Myeloproliferative disease
Myelophthisis
Hypersplenism
Lead poisoning
Leukemias

## Feline Immunodeficiency Virus Testing

Presence of antibody-indicates infection—cats never clear
  infection
  False-positive
    Interference by vaccination in tests that do not con-
      tain the gp40 capture antigen. Presence of maternal
      antibody in kittens of infected or vaccinated queens
      (detectable up to 6 months of age)
  False-negative
    Acute infection up to 8 weeks required for antibody
      production
Confirmatory testing

Western blot antibody test
Confirmatory test of choice for antibody
Higher sensitivity and specificity than ELISA
Polymerase chain reaction (detection of proviral DNA)
Can differentiate between vaccinated and infected cat
Not very sensitive or specific

## Folate

*Normal Range*
Feline: 9.7–21.6 ng/mL
Canine: 7.7–24.4 ng/mL
Usually performed in conjunction with serum cobalamin and
trypsinlike immunoreactivity

*Elevated in:*
exocrine pancreatic insufficiency, small intestinal bacterial
overgrowth (intestinal dysbiosis), dietary supplementation

*Decreased in:*
small intestinal mucosal disease, antibiotics depleting intestinal
flora

## Fructosamine

*Normal Range*
Feline and canine: 175–400 µmol/L
Single sample test that assays mean blood glucose over the
previous 1–3 weeks

*Elevated:*
>500 µmol/L indicates poor glycemic control (hyperglycemia)
Declining or within normal range: indicates improving or
adequate glycemic control

*Decreased to below lower end of reference range
(<300 µmol/L):*
suggests that patient has experienced significant periods of
hypoglycemia over past 1–3 weeks, also hypoalbuminemia/
hypoproteinemia may falsely lower fructosamine
Values within normal range with PU/PD (polyuria/polydipsia)
and polyphagia: suggestive of Somogyi phenomenon

*Note: Fructosamine values should not be used to make specific
adjustments in insulin dosage.*

## Gamma Glutamyltransferase (GGT)

*Normal Range*
Feline: 1–4 U/L
Canine: 1–6 U/L

*Elevated:*
cholestasis—GGT mirrors alkaline phosphatase (intrahepatic, extrahepatic), drugs (dogs [glucocorticoids]), anticonvulsants (phenobarbital, primidone), hepatocellular disease (generally slight increase)

> Note: *Cats with hepatic lipidosis tend to have normal to mildly elevated GGT but greatly elevated alkaline phosphatase levels.*

*Decreased:*
spurious (e.g., laboratory error, lipemic sample), hemolysis

## Globulin

*Normal Range*
Feline: 2.3–5.3 g/dL
Canine: 1.6–3.6 g/dL

*Elevated in:*
dehydration (albumin and total protein also elevated); infection (polyclonal gammopathy; chronic pyoderma, pyometra, chronic periodontitis, FIP, bacterial endocarditis, brucellosis, FIV, FeLV, ehrlichiosis [may cause polyclonal or monoclonal gammopathy], heartworm disease, leishmaniasis [may cause polyclonal or monoclonal gammopathy], systemic mycoses, chronic pneumonia, bartonellosis, *Mycoplasma haemofelis* infection, Chagas disease, babesiosis); immune-mediated disease (polyclonal gammopathy); neoplasia (polyclonal gammopathy [necrotic or draining tumors, lymphomas, mast cell tumors]); neoplasia (monoclonal gammopathy [multiple myeloma, chronic lymphocytic leukemia, lymphoma]); cutaneous amyloidosis; idiopathic monoclonal gammopathy

## Glucose

*Normal Range*
Feline: 64–170 mg/dL
Canine: 70–138 mg/dL

*Elevated (hyperglycemia) in:*

diabetes mellitus, stress (cats), hyperadrenocorticism, pancreatitis, drugs (glucocorticoids, progestogens, megestrol acetate, thiazide diuretics), parenteral nutrition, dextrose-containing fluids, postprandial, acromegaly (cats), diestrus (bitch), pheochromocytoma (dogs), exocrine pancreatic neoplasia, renal insufficiency, head trauma

*Decreased (hypoglycemia) in:*

depatic insufficiency (portosystemic shunts, chronic fibrosis, cirrhosis); sepsis; prolonged sample storage; iatrogenic (insulin therapy, sulfonylurea therapy); toxicity (ethanol ingestion, ethylene glycol, xylitol, oleander); β-cell tumor (insulinoma); extrapancreatic neoplasia (hepatocellular carcinoma or hepatoma, leiomyosarcoma or leiomyoma, hemangiosarcoma, carcinoma [mammary, salivary, pulmonary], leukemia, plasmacytoma, melanoma); hypoadrenocorticism; hypopituitarism; idiopathic hypoglycemia (neonatal hypoglycemia, juvenile hypoglycemia [Toy breeds], hunting dog hypoglycemia); renal failure; exocrine pancreatic neoplasia; glycogen storage diseases; severe polycythemia; prolonged starvation; laboratory error

## Glucose Tolerance Test

May be used to differentiate type 1 (insulin-dependent) from type 2 (non-insulin-dependent) diabetes mellitus in cats (all dogs are considered to have type 1); results inconsistent; not usually done

## Glycated (Glycosylated) Hemoglobin

Assays measure mean blood glucose over the lifespan of erythrocytes (3–4 months); in dogs, values between 4% and 6% are associated with adequate glycemic control; used less often than fructosamine.

## Heartworm Antibody, Feline

Should be interpreted in conjunction with a feline heartworm antigen test

Should be interpreted in light of clinical, clinicopathologic, and radiographic signs

A negative test suggests no exposure to *Dirofilaria immitis* and helps to rule out.

A positive test supports prior exposure but does not confirm active infection.

## Heartworm Antigen, Canine

A negative test implies no infection.

A positive test supports active infection.

Positive tests should be confirmed by using a different manufacturer's antigen or by demonstrating circulating microfilaria.

A sample hemolysis may cause a false-positive result.

A low worm burden, only male worms present, or immature infestations may cause a false-negative result.

The results may remain positive for up to 16 weeks after successful adulticide therapy.

## Heartworm Antigen, Feline

Should be interpreted in conjunction with a feline heartworm antibody test

Negative test should be recorded as "no antigen detected" (NAD), not negative.

Positive test is highly specific; infection is likely.

Should be interpreted in light of clinical, clinicopathologic, and radiographic signs

Sample hemolysis may cause false-positive results.

Low worm burden or male unisex infection will cause false-negative results.

## Hematocrit (PCV)

*Normal Range*
Feline: 29%–48%
Canine: 36%–60%

*Increased in:*
dehydration (total protein also increased), polycythemia, splenic contracture, hypoxemia

*Decreased in:*
anemia (for more detailed list, see Erythrocyte Count); color of plasma in spun-down hematocrit tube can help determine if icterus (yellow) or intravascular hemolysis (red) is present; buffy coat: may see microfilaria if patient has heartworm disease; mast cells in systemic mastocytosis

## Hemoglobin

Hemoglobin concentrations are usually proportional to hematocrit except in rare cases where hemoglobin synthesis defects stimulate polycythemia

## Hemolysis, Prevention in Laboratory Samples

### Steps to Prevent Hemolysis

Fasted patient: lipemia increases red cell fragility

Minimize negative pressure (may cause vein to flutter against needle, crushing red cells)

Reposition needle deeper, or slightly rotate to move bevel of needle away from vessel wall

Resist tendency to increase vacuum by using more negative force; "milk" the vein

Use vacuum tubes and needles instead of syringes

Remove needle and specimen tube stopper, and transfer sample directly into open tube

Aspirate small amount of air from tube to reestablish negative pressure to prevent tops from coming off in transit

Avoid small-diameter needles for sample collection

Promptly separate serum from clot and store properly

Avoid delays in sample transport and analysis, and avoid extremes of temperature

## Immunoassays

### Assays That Detect All Immunoglobulins to a Specific Antigen in a Serum Sample

#### COMPLEMENT FIXATION

Hemagglutination inhibition

Serum neutralization

Agglutination assay

Agar gel immunodiffusion

Indirect fluorescent antibody

### Assays That May Be Used to Detect Specific Immunoglobulins (IgG, IgM, IgA) to Antigens in a Serum Sample

#### ENZYME-LINKED IMMUNOSORBENT ASSAY (ELISA)

Western blot immunoassay

IgM usually first immunoglobulin produced; may indicate recent infection and more likely to be active infection rather than just previous exposure

Production of immunoglobulin shifts to IgG and/or IgA in days to weeks; indicates more chronic infection and possibly exposure without active disease.

Demonstrating a rising titer with paired samples may be necessary to document active infection.

## Insulin

*Normal Range*
Feline and canine: 15–35 µIU/mL

*Elevated:*
expected response to hyperglycemia; normal or elevated insulin concentration in the presence of hypoglycemia is supportive of insulinoma (pancreatic islet beta-cell neoplasia); also may be elevated with insulin therapy or leiomyosarcoma

*Decreased:*
decreased insulin levels are not a reliable indicator of diabetes mellitus; patients with insulin-dependent diabetes mellitus (IDDM) should have low insulin and high glucose levels; insulin levels in non–insulin-dependent diabetes mellitus (NIDDM) are variable.

## Iron-Binding Capacity (Total, TIBC)/Ferritin

Decreased TIBC and decreased ferritin: chronic (not acute) blood loss (intestinal ulceration, hookworm anemia, bleeding from neoplasia, hepatic insufficiency, protein-losing enteropathy or nephropathy, etc.)
TIBC normal to increased, ferritin decreased: iron deficiency
TIBC normal to low, ferritin normal to high: anemia of chronic inflammatory disease

## Joint Fluid (Arthrocentesis)

### Gross Appearance

Evaluate for turbidity (cloudiness), viscosity (does it form a long string when allowed to drip from a needle?), and color (clear, red or hemorrhagic, yellow); yellow color (xanthochromia) may indicate previous hemorrhage, degenerative, traumatic, or inflammatory disease

### Gross Appearance, Microscopic Examination/Cytologic Evaluation

*NORMAL*
Straw-colored, clear, viscous, firm mucin clot test
1–3 mononuclear cells per high-power field (hpf)
Large and small mononuclear cells with numerous vacuoles and granules; less than 10% are neutrophils (<1 neutrophil/500 erythrocytes if blood contamination has occurred)

## HEMARTHROSIS

Bloody or xanthochromic, turbid, reduced viscosity, normal to slightly friable mucin clot test

Hemosiderin-laden macrophage, erythrophagia, moderate neutrophils

## CHRONIC DEGENERATIVE JOINT DISEASE

Light yellow, clear to slightly turbid, viscous, normal firm mucin clot

0%–20% neutrophils, few to moderate lymphocytes and macrophages

### *Immune-Mediated Joint Disease (Nonerosive)*

Yellow to blood-tinged, slight to moderate turbidity, reduced viscosity, friable mucin clot test

15%–95% neutrophils, few to moderate lymphocytes, synoviocytes, macrophages

### Traumatic

Straw-colored to blood-tinged, slight to moderate turbidity, normal to slightly turbid, normal to slightly friable mucin clot test

Variable neutrophils

May see hemorrhage

### Septic

Yellow to blood-tinged to bloody, turbid to purulent, reduced viscosity, friable mucin clot test

90%–99% neutrophils

May see microorganisms within cells

Toxic changes in neutrophils

### Rheumatoid Arthritis (Erosive)

Yellow to blood-tinged, turbid, reduced viscosity, friable mucin clot test

20%–80% neutrophils

SLE-induced polyarthritis: may see LE cells

## Lactate

*Normal Range*

Feline: 0.5–2.0 mmol/L

Canine: 0.3–2.5 mmol/L

## Causes of Lactic Acidosis in Veterinary Medicine

Markedly elevated lactate values are associated with a poor prognosis in critical care settings

### TYPE A (MECHANISM: TISSUE HYPOXIA OR HYPOPERFUSION)

Decreased $O_2$ delivery

- Anemia
- Shock (cardiogenic, septic, hypovolemic)
- Regional hypoperfusion
- Global hypoperfusion
- Carbon monoxide intoxication

Increased $O_2$ demand

- Exercise
- Seizures
- Uncontrolled shivering

## TYPE B1 (MECHANISM: DECREASED LACTATE CLEARANCE)

Hepatic disease
Diabetes mellitus
Sepsis, systemic inflammatory response syndrome (SIRS)
Renal failure
Hyperthyroidism
Neoplasia
Alkalosis

## TYPE B2 (MECHANISM: DRUGS OR TOXINS THAT INTERFERE WITH OXIDATIVE PHOSPHORYLATION)

Ethylene glycol
Propylene glycol
Catecholamines
Carbon monoxide
Bicarbonate
Salicylates
Acetaminophen
Others (cyanide, strychnine, nitroprusside, halothane, terbutaline, activated charcoal)

## TYPE B3 (MECHANISM: MITOCHONDRIAL DEFECTS)

Mitochondrial myopathies (inborn and acquired)

## D-LACTIC ACIDOSIS (MECHANISM: PRODUCTION OF D-LACTATE FROM BACTERIAL GLUCOSE METABOLISM OR ALTERNATIVE METABOLIC PATHWAYS)

Diabetes mellitus
Small intestinal bacterial overgrowth
Exocrine pancreatic insufficiency
Propylene glycol toxicosis

## Lipase

*Normal Range*
Feline: 10–450 U/L
Canine: 77–695 U/L

*Elevated in:*
Most often seen with acute pancreatitis, pancreatic necrosis, pancreatic neoplasia, enteritis, renal disease, hepatic disease, glucocorticoids; rarely elevated with certain neoplasms in the absence of pancreatitis

*Note:* Not very sensitive or specific for pancreatic disease

## Lymphocyte Count

*Normal Range*
Feline: 1200–8000 cells/μL
Canine: 690–4500 cells/μL

*Elevated (lymphocytosis)*
physiologic or epinephrine induced, postvaccination, leukemia (lymphocytic, lymphoblastic), chronic antigenic stimulation (e.g., chronic infection, viremia, immune-mediated, inflammatory bowel disease, cholangiohepatitis, ehrlichiosis, Chagas disease, babesiosis, leishmaniasis, hypoadrenocorticism)

*Decreased (lymphopenia)*
corticosteroid- or stress induced; chemotherapy; immunodeficiency (FeLV, FIV); loss of lymph (chylothorax, lymphangiectasia); viral disease (FeLV/FIV, FIP, parvovirus, canine distemper, canine infectious hepatitis)

## Magnesium (Mg)

*Normal Range*
Feline: 1.1–2.3 mEq/L
Canine: 1.2–1.9 mEq/L

*Increased in:*
renal failure or insufficiency, excessive oral intake (antacids, laxatives), excessive parenteral administration, angiotensin-converting enzyme (ACE) inhibitors, spironolactone

*Decreased:*
dietary, GI (malabsorption, chronic diarrhea, pancreatitis, cholestatic liver disease), renal (glomerular disease, tubular disease, postobstructive diuresis, prolonged intravenous fluids, diuretics, digitalis administration, hypercalcemia, hypokalemia), endocrine (diabetic ketoacidosis, hyperthyroidism, primary hyperparathyroidism, primary hyperaldosteronism), multiple endocrine disorders, sepsis, blood transfusion, parenteral

nutrition, hypothermia, dialysis, drugs (diuretics, amphotericin B, insulin, glucose, amino acids)

## Mean Corpuscular Volume (MCV)

**Normal Range**
Feline: 37–61 fL
Canine: 58–79 fL

**Elevated (macrocytosis) in:**
regeneration, FeLV, FIV, breed-related characteristics (Poodles), dyserythropoiesis (bone marrow disease), sample artifact (swelling of RBCs secondary to prolonged storage in EDTA tubes)

**Decreased (microcytosis) in:**
iron deficiency, portosystemic shunt, polycythemia, breed-related characteristics (Akita, Shar-Pei, Shiba Inu)

## Methemoglobinemia

Methemoglobin is the form of hemoglobin in which the heme iron has been oxidized from ferrous ($Fe^{2+}$) to ferric ($Fe^{3+}$) and is rendered unable to bind and transport oxygen.

Methemoglobinemia is seen in oxidative damage-induced hemolytic anemias (e.g., nitrite, copper, acetaminophen, benzocaine, phenazopyridine, zinc) and with rare inherited erythrocyte disorders.

## Methods of Sample Collection for Cytology

### Fine-Needle Biopsy (Aspiration or Nonaspiration Method)

Surface masses
Internal masses
Lymph nodes
Internal organs
Fluid collection

### Impression Smear

Exudative cutaneous lesions
Preparation of cytology samples from biopsy specimens

### Scraping

Flat cutaneous lesions not amenable to fine-needle biopsy
Preparation of cytologic samples from poorly exfoliative biopsy specimens

## Swab

Vaginal smears
Fistulous tracts
Otic swabs
Nasal, conjunctival swabs

## Microfilaria Testing

Direct examination of a drop of blood under a microscope or examination of the buffy coat for microfilaria are insensitive testing methods.

The modified Knott test is the preferred concentration technique for determining the absence or presence of microfilaria. It also allows for measuring worm dimensions to differentiate *Dirofilaria immitis* from *Acanthocheilonema* (formerly *Dipetalonema*) filarial species.

Cats are seldom microfilaremic. Chances of finding microfilaria are improved with concentrating tests like the modified Knott test.

## MiraVista Fungal Testing

With systemic fungal diseases, fungal agents may shed specific structural antigens into body cavity fluids such as serum, urine, CSF, BAL fluid. Urine is most often tested.

Tests include assays for *Aspergillus* spp, *Blastomyces dermatitidis, Coccidioides* spp, *Cryptococcus neoformans, and Histoplasma capsulatum.*

False-positive and -negative results may occur so best interpreted with cytologic or histopathologic identification of fungal elements.

## Monocyte Count

### Normal Range
Feline: 0–600 cells/μL
Canine: 0–840 cells/μL

### Elevated (monocytosis) in:
infection (pyometra, abscess, peritonitis, pyothorax, osteomyelitis, prostatitis, *Mycoplasma haemofelis*, blastomycosis, histoplasmosis, *Cryptococcus*, Coccidioides, heartworm disease, other bacteria [e.g., nocardiosis, actinomycosis, mycobacteriosis]); stress or corticosteroid induced; immune-mediated disease (hemolytic anemia, dermatitis, polyarthritis); trauma with severe crushing injury; hemorrhage into tissues or body cavities; neoplasia (tumor necrosis, lymphoma, myelodysplastic

disorders, leukemias, myelomonocytic leukemia, monocytic leukemia, myelogenous leukemia, hemophagic histiocytic sarcoma)

## Myoglobinuria

Brown to dark-red urine with an absence of RBCs in urine sediment and a positive test for occult blood; seen with generalized muscle disease

## Neutrophil Count

### Normal Range
Feline: 2500–8500 cells/µL
Canine: 2060–10,600 cells/µL

### Elevated (neutrophilia):
Increased production (infection [bacterial, systemic mycoses, protozoal], inflammation [immune-mediated disease, neoplasia, tissue trauma, tissue necrosis]); demargination (stress, hyperadrenocorticism, glucocorticoids); metabolic (uremia, diabetic ketoacidosis); associated with regenerative anemia (hemolytic anemia, hemorrhagic anemia); chronic granulocytic leukemia

### Decreased (neutropenia):
Decreased production (myelophthisis [myeloproliferative disease, lymphoproliferative disease, metastatic neoplasia], myelofibrosis, drug-induced [chemotherapeutics, griseofulvin, chloramphenicol, trimethoprim-sulfa, azathioprine, estrogen, phenylbutazone, phenobarbital], infectious [parvovirus, ehrlichiosis, FIV, FeLV {aplastic anemia, myelodysplasia, panleukopenia-like syndrome}], hypersplenism, idiopathic hypoplasia/aplasia [cyclic neutropenia, immune-mediated]); increased consumption (bacteremia/septicemia, severe systemic infection, endotoxemia); hypoadrenocorticism; margination

## NT-proBNP

N-terminal pro-B-type natriuretic peptide
Circulating biomarker for cardiac disease in dogs and cats

### Elevated in
- Increased intracardiac hydrostatic pressure
- Slight increase with pulmonary disease or pulmonary hypertension
- Slight increase with prerenal or renal azotemia

May help differentiate dyspneic patients with cardiogenic pulmonary edema from those with noncardiac disease

## Osmolality

Plasma osmolality is expected to be decreased in primary polydipsia (psychogenic polydipsia); diabetic ketoacidosis; azotemia; hypernatremia; hyperglycemia; and intoxication with ethylene glycol, ethanol, or methanol.

Plasma osmolality is expected to be increased in primary polyuria (DI).

There may be considerable overlap in values of primary polyuria and polydipsia. However, osmolality of <280 mOsm/kg suggests psychogenic polydipsia, whereas osmolality of >280 mOsm/kg suggests central DI, nephrogenic DI, or psychogenic polydipsia.

## Packed Cell Volume

See Hematocrit

## Pancreatic Lipase Immunoreactivity (PLI)

*Normal Range*

*TRYPSINOGEN-LIKE IMMUNOREACTIVITY*
Feline: 12.0–82.0 µg/L
Canine: 5.7–45.2.0 µg/L

*PANCREATIC LIPASE IMMUNOREACTIVITY*
Feline: 0.1–3.5 µg/L
Canine: 0–200 µg/L

Low TLI values (<2.5 µg/L for dogs and <8.0 µg/L for cats) are diagnostic for exocrine pancreatic insufficiency; values between 2.5 and 5.0 µg/L for dogs and 8.0 and 12.0 µg/L for cats are considered equivocal, and the assay should be repeated in 1 month.

High values for TLI are supportive of a diagnosis of acute or chronic pancreatitis.

Elevated values for PLI (>12 µg/L for cats and >400 µg/L for dogs) are consistent with a diagnosis of pancreatitis.

Patients must be fasted at least 12 hours.

*Note: These tests are species specific, and samples must be labeled "dog" or "cat" so that the test can be performed correctly.*

## Parathyroid Hormone (PTH)/Ionized Calcium

*Normal Range*

*PARATHYROID HORMONE*
Feline: 0.0–40.0 pg/mL
Canine: 20.0–130.0 pg/mL

*IONIZED CALCIUM*
Feline: 1.16–1.34 mmol/L
Canine: 1.24–1.43 mmol/L

*Elevated in:*
primary hyperparathyroidism (elevated ionized calcium and mid-to-high elevated PTH), renal or nutritional secondary hyperparathyroidism (normal or decreased ionized calcium and elevated PTH), hypercalcemia of malignancy, vitamin D toxicity, granulomatous inflammatory disease

*Decreased in:*
primary hypoparathyroidism (decreased ionized calcium and low or low-to-normal PTH)

## Parathyroid Hormone-Related Protein (PTHrP)

*Increased in*
Humoral hypercalcemia of malignancy
- T-cell lymphoma
- Anal sac apocrine gland adenocarcinoma
- Parathyroid adenoma
- Malignant melanoma
- Squamous cell carcinoma
- Mammary adenocarcinoma
- Thyroid carcinoma
- Bronchoalveolar carcinoma
- Multiple myeloma

## Phosphorus (P)

*Normal Range*
Feline: 2.4–8.2 mg/dL
Canine: 2.5–6.0 mg/dL

*Elevated in:*
young, growing animal; reduced glomerular filtration rate (GFR, acute renal failure [ARF], chronic renal failure); postrenal obstruction, primary hypoparathyroidism, nutritional secondary hyperparathyroidism, hyperthyroidism, acromegaly, hemolysis, intoxication (hypervitaminosis D, jasmine ingestion);

dietary excess; metabolic acidosis; iatrogenic (phosphate enemas, parenteral administration); osteolysis; osteolytic neoplasia; rhabdomyolysis; tumor cell lysis syndrome; sample hemolysis/delayed serum separation

*Decreased in:*
primary hyperparathyroidism (also see Increased Calcium); nutritional secondary hyperparathyroidism; renal tubular acidosis; vomiting/diarrhea; neoplasia (PTH-like hormone, C-cell thyroid tumors); insulin therapy; diabetic ketoacidosis; Fanconi syndrome; dietary deficiency; decrease intestinal absorption; eclampsia; hyperadrenocorticism; vitamin D deficiency; hyperaldosteronism; aggressive fluid therapy; bicarbonate administration; respiratory or metabolic acidosis

## PIVKA

Proteins induced by vitamin K absence or antagonism
Inactive precursor coagulation proteins accumulate in the
    blood when vitamin K is absent or inhibited.

*Increased in*
decreased vitamin K: neonate born to malnourished mother,
    prolonged anorexia
malabsorption of vitamin K: cholestasis, infiltrative bowel
    disease
vitamin K antagonism: anticoagulant rodenticides, therapeutic
    warfarin

## Platelet Count

*Normal Range*
Feline: 200–500×103/μL
Canine: 170–400×10$^3$/μL

*Elevated in:*
neoplasia (essential thrombocytosis, acute megakaryocytic leukemia); increased production (inflammation, rebound thrombocytosis, iron deficiency); polycythemia vera; hyperadrenocorticism; immune-mediated hemolytic anemia

*Decreased (see Thrombocytopenia p. 186):*
decreased production (infectious [retroviruses: FIV, FeLV; *Ehrlichia*, infiltrative bone marrow disease]); increased destruction (immune-mediated thrombocytopenia, *Babesia, Anaplasma platys*); sequestration (hypersplenism); increased consumption (hemorrhage, DIC, vasculitis); breed idiosyncrasy (Cavalier King Charles Spaniels [macrothrombocytes], Greyhounds)

## Polymerase Chain Reaction

PCR amplifies small quantities of DNA to detectable levels.

Can also be used to detect RNA with a reverse transcriptase step (RT-PCR)

In general, PCR is more sensitive than cytologic, serologic, or histopathologic techniques and is comparable to culture.

PCR is of great benefit for demonstration of infectious agents, especially if the organism is difficult to culture or cannot be cultured.

Specificity can be quite high, depending on the primers used in the reaction. For example, primers can be designed to detect one bacterial genus but not others. Primers can also be designed to identify one species (e.g., all *Ehrlichia* spp. or only *E. canis*).

False-positive if sample is contaminated during collection or in laboratory

False-negative if sample is handled inappropriately

## Potassium (K)

*Normal Range*
Feline: 3.4–5.6 g/dL
Canine: 3.6–5.5 g/dL

*Elevated in:*
renal failure (distal renal tubular acidosis, oliguric/anuric); postrenal (obstruction, ruptured bladder); hypoadrenocorticism; acidosis (diabetic ketoacidosis); GI (trichuriasis, salmonellosis, perforated duodenal ulcer); chylothorax with repeated pleural fluid drainage; massive muscle trauma; postischemic reperfusion; dehydration; hypoaldosteronism; drugs (potassium-sparing diuretics, ACE inhibitors, propranolol); thrombocytosis; severe leukocytosis (>100,000/µL); hemolysis in breed with high RBC potassium concentration (Akita, English Springer Spaniel, neonates, individuals); hyperkalemic periodic paralysis

*Decreased in:*
alkalosis; dietary deficiency (feline); potassium-free fluids; bicarbonate administration; drugs (penicillins, amphotericin B, loop diuretics, thiazide diuretics); GI fluid loss (vomiting and diarrhea, potassium rich); hyperadrenocorticism; hyperaldosteronism; insulin therapy; diuresis caused by diabetic ketoacidosis; renal (postobstructive diuresis, renal tubular acidosis, dialysis); hypokalemic periodic paralysis (Burmese cat, American Pit Bull Terrier); renal failure (chronic polyuria); total parenteral nutrition

## Protein Electrophoresis

*Elevated in:*
increased alpha globulin: acute inflammation, nephrotic syndrome, corticosteroids
increased beta globulin: acute inflammation, nephrotic syndrome, liver disease, immune responses, neoplasia
increased gamma globulins: immune stimulation, neoplasia
polyclonal gammopathy: inflammation, infection, immune-
mediated disease, liver disease, neoplasia (neoplasia more
commonly monoclonal)
monoclonal gammopathy: multiple myeloma, B-cell lymphoma, lymphocytic leukemia, inflammatory, infection
(ehrlichiosis, feline infectious peritonitis, leishmaniasis,
feline stomatitis, lymphoplasmacytic enterocolitis)

*Decreased in:*
decreased albumin: acute-phase response, glomerular disease,
liver disease, starvation, cachexia
decreased albumin and globulin: GI disease (protein-losing
enteropathy), blood loss, sequestration in body cavity effusions,
severe exudative skin disease, excess fluid therapy, excess water
intake
decreased globulins: failure of passive transfer, inherited or
acquired immunodeficiency

## Protein, Total (TP)

*Normal Range*
Feline: 5.2–8.8 g/dL
Canine: 5.0–7.4 g/dL

*Elevated in:*
dehydration (albumin and globulin increased); hyperglobulinemia (chronic inflammation, infection, neoplasia [e.g., multiple
myeloma]); spurious (hemolysis, lipemia)

*Decreased in:*
hemorrhage, hypoalbuminemia, liver failure, external plasma
loss, GI fluid loss, malassimilation, starvation, overhydration,
glomerular loss, tumor cachexia

## Prothrombin Time (PT)

*Normal Range*
Feline: 6–11 seconds
Canine: 6–12 seconds

Determines abnormalities in the extrinsic coagulation pathway

Prolonged with deficiencies of factors II, VII, and X

Becomes prolonged before any changes seen in ACT or activated partial thromboplastin time (aPTT)

Prolonged with DIC, acquired vitamin K deficiency (rodenticide poisoning), bile insufficiency, and liver failure

## Red Blood Cell Count

See Erythrocyte Count

## Reticulocyte Count

Elevated reticulocyte count is the best indicator of effective erythropoiesis.

*Step 1:* Multiply percent reticulocytes by red cell count to determine absolute quantity

*Step 2:* Correct for reduced red cell mass; multiply absolute reticulocytes by patient's hematocrit divided by mean species hematocrit to obtain the number of reticulocytes per milliliter

*Step 3:* Correct for the effect of erythropoietin on the bone marrow reticulocyte release; divide the number of reticulocytes per milliliter by average number of days that a reticulocyte circulates in peripheral blood at that patient's hematocrit to obtain a corrected absolute reticulocyte count

A corrected absolute reticulocyte count of less than 105,000/mL is indicative of a nonregenerative anemia, whereas strongly regenerative anemias will have a reticulocyte count of greater than 150,000/mL.

Reticulocytosis without anemia can be linked to drug therapy (glucocorticoids, NSAIDs) or dietary supplements (glucosamine, omega-3 fatty acids) that stimulate erythropoiesis.

## Sodium (Na)

***Normal Range***
Feline: 145–158 mEq/L
Canine: 139–154 mEq/L

***Elevated in:***
dehydration; renal failure; GI fluid loss (Na$^+$-poor) (vomiting, diarrhea); insensible fluid loss (panting, high ambient

temperature, fever); third space loss (i.e., pancreatitis, peritonitis); cutaneous loss (e.g., burns); decreased water intake (limited access to water, primary adipsia); hyperaldosteronemia; increased salt intake (oral, intravenous); toxicosis (paintball ingestion, phosphate enema), spurious (evaporation of serum sample)

*Decreased in:*
hypoadrenocorticism; GI fluid loss ($Na^+$-rich) (vomiting, diarrhea); severe liver disease; hookworms; renal failure (polyuric); nephrotic syndrome causing effusion; chronic effusions; diuretics; hypotonic fluids; diabetes mellitus; mannitol infusion; burns; excess antidiuretic hormone (ADH); diet (severe sodium restriction); antidiuretic drugs (e.g., vincristine, cyclophosphamide, nonsteroidal antiinflammatory drugs [NSAIDs]); myxedema coma of hypothyroidism; psychogenic polydipsia; spurious (hyperlipidemia, marked hyperproteinemia)

## Specific Gravity

*Normal*
Feline: 1.025–1.060 (high normal range values may be a risk factor for feline lower urinary tract disease [FLUTD])
Canine: 1.020–1.050

*ISOSTHENURIA (1.008–1.012)*
Renal failure
Rare cases of polydipsia

*HYPOSTHENURIA (<1.008)*
Polydipsia/polyuria (e.g., hyperthyroidism, hypercalcemia, hypokalemia, hepatic failure, psychogenic)
DI

## Chemical Properties

### PH

*Normal*
5.5–7.5 (feline and canine)
*Causes of acidic urine:* meat-based diet; administration of acidifying agents (e.g., D,L-methionine, $NH_4Cl$); metabolic acidosis; respiratory acidosis; protein catabolic states; severe vomiting with chloride depletion
*Causes of alkaline urine:* vegetable-based diet; administration of alkalinizing agents (e.g., $NaHCO_3$, citrate); urinary

tract infection by urease-producing bacteria; postprandial alkaline tide; metabolic alkalosis; respiratory alkalosis; renal tubular acidosis (distal tubule)

### PROTEIN

*Normal*

0–30 mg/dL

Must be interpreted in light of urine specific gravity

Commonly used dipsticks are more sensitive to albumin than globulin.

Increased with glomerular or inflammatory disease

#### GLUCOSE

Appears in urine if the renal threshold is exceeded

Diabetes mellitus, stress (especially in cats), infusion of dextrose-containing fluids, pheochromocytoma, proximal renal tubular diseases (aminoglycoside toxicity, ARF, Fanconi syndrome, primary renal glucosuria)

#### KETONES

Test pad measures acetoacetate and acetone but not beta-hydroxybutyrate, which is responsible for acidosis.

*Elevated in:*

Diabetic ketoacidosis, starvation, prolonged fasting, glycogen storage disease, low-carbohydrate diet, persistent fever, persistent hypoglycemia

#### OCCULT BLOOD

Does not differentiate among erythrocytes (RBCs), hemoglobin, and myoglobin

Always interpreted in light of urine sediment (evaluation for RBCs)

Erythrocytes—hematuria

Hemoglobin—hemolysis

Myoglobin—rhabdomyolysis

#### BILIRUBIN

Detectable in urine before it is elevated in serum

May be found in trace amounts in concentrated samples, especially in intact males

Bilirubinuria seen in hemolysis, liver disease, extrahepatic obstruction, fever, starvation.

#### UROBILINOGEN

Presence indicates normal enterohepatic bilirubin circulation.

## Urinary Sediment Examination

### RED BLOOD CELLS

Normally, zero to occasional RBCs; excessive RBCs termed *hematuria* (see p. 47)

### WHITE BLOOD CELLS

Normally, zero to occasional WBCs

Excessive WBCs termed *pyuria;* indicates urinary tract infection but does not localize the site of infection.

### EPITHELIAL CELLS

Squamous and transitional cells; little diagnostic significance

Increased transitional cells may be seen with infection, neoplasia, and irritation of the urinary tract

### CASTS

Cylindrical molds of renal tubules composed of aggregated proteins or cells that localize disease to the kidney

Occasional hyaline or granular casts may be normal; cellular casts are always abnormal

*Hyaline Casts*

Protein precipitates (Tamm–Horsfall mucoprotein and albumin); seen with proteinuric renal disease (glomerulonephritis, amyloidosis), small numbers with fever and exercise

*Granular Casts*

Degeneration of cells in casts or precipitation of filtered plasma proteins; suggest ischemic or nephrotoxic renal tubular injury

*Cellular Casts*

WBC casts (pyelonephritis), RBC casts (fragile, rare in dogs and cats), renal epithelial cell casts (acute tubular necrosis or pyelonephritis)

*Fatty Casts*

Lipid granules (nephrotic syndrome or diabetes mellitus)

*Waxy Casts*

Final stage of degeneration of granular casts (suggest intrarenal stasis)

### ORGANISMS

Small numbers of bacteria may contaminate voided or catheterized samples, but usually not enough to be seen in urine sediment unless sample is allowed to incubate. Presence of large numbers of bacteria in sediment suggests urinary tract infection. Yeast and fungal hyphae usually are contaminants.

## CRYSTALS

Usually of little diagnostic value; may be found in normal urine

Acidic urine may contain urate, calcium oxalate, and cystine crystals.

Alkaline urine may contain struvite, calcium phosphate, calcium carbonate, amorphous phosphate, and ammonium biurate crystals.

Bilirubin crystals may be seen with concentrated samples or with bilirubinuria.

Urate crystals may be seen in Dalmatians and with liver disease or portosystemic shunts.

Struvite crystals are seen in cats with idiopathic lower urinary tract disease, dogs and cats with struvite urolithiasis.

Calcium oxalate in oliguric ARF suggests ethylene glycol intoxication.

Cystine crystals, when abnormal, suggest cystinuria.

## OTHER FINDINGS IN SEDIMENT

Sperm in intact male dogs

Parasite ova; *Dioctophyma renale, Capillaria plica*

Microfilariae

Lipid droplets (diabetes mellitus, nephrotic syndrome, in cats with degeneration of lipid-laden tubular cells)

## COMMON BACTERIA SEEN IN URINARY TRACT INFECTIONS

*E. coli*

*Proteus* spp.

*Staphylococcus* spp.

*Pasteurella multocida*

*Enterobacter* spp.

*Klebsiella* spp.

*Pseudomonas aeruginosa*

## Symmetric Dimethylarginine (SDMA) Assay

SDMA is a renal biomarker specific to kidney function. SDMA increases with as little as 25% loss of kidney function, making it more reliable in both acute or active kidney injury and chronic kidney disease. Creatinine cannot identify kidney issues until almost 75% of kidney function is lost.

*Normal Range*
Feline 0–14 µg/dL
Canine 0–14 µg/dL (0–16 µg/dL in puppies)

*Elevated in:*
impaired glomerular filtration (prerenal, renal, and postrenal causes)

## Synovial Fluid Analysis

*Normal synovial fluid:*
- Colorless to pale yellow
- Viscous
- High mucin (hyaluronic acid) content
- Does not clot
- RBCs absent, nucleated cells 500-3000 μL (synoviocytes and macrophages predominate)
- Protein content 1.8-4.8 g/dL

*Abnormal synovial fluid:*
Increased erythrocytes: iatrogenic blood contamination, hemarthrosis
Increased nucleated cell count:
- Mononuclear cells predominate in degenerative and inflammatory arthropathies
  - Trauma
  - Osteoarthrosis
  - Osteochondritis dessicans
  - Aseptic necrosis of the femoral head (Legg-Calve-Perthes disease
- Neutrophils predominate in inflammatory arthropathies
  - Bacterial-monoarticular due to penetrating trauma
  - Systemic bacterial
  - Tick-borne disease
  - Fungal infection
  - Viral infection
  - Mycoplasmal infection
  - Immune-mediated polyarthritis
  - Chronic progressive polyarthritis in cats

## Thoracentesis Fluid

### Pyothorax (Septic)

Extremely high nucleated cell counts (>50,000/μL), protein >3.0 g/dL
Primarily degenerate neutrophils and macrophages
Bacteria seen in WBCs
Penetrating wounds, foreign body (grass awns), extension of bacterial pneumonia or discospondylitis, postoperative infection

## Nonseptic

Moderate nucleated cell counts (>5000/µL)

Neutrophils, macrophages, eosinophils, lymphocytes

FIP, neoplasia, diaphragmatic hernia, lung lobe torsion

## Chylous Effusion

Low-to-moderate nucleated cell counts (400–10,000/µL)

Predominant cell type is small lymphocyte; also neutrophils and macrophages

Triglyceride concentration of pleural fluid is greater than that of serum

Idiopathic

Congenital

Secondary to neoplasia, trauma, cardiac disease, fungal granuloma, pericardial disease, dirofilariasis, lung lobe torsion, diaphragmatic hernia, pericardial diaphragmatic hernia, vena caval thrombosis

## Hemorrhagic Effusion

Trauma

Coagulopathy

Neoplasia

Lung lobe torsion

Rupture of vessels associated with parasitic infection (*Spirocerca lupi, Dirofilaria immitis*)

## Transudates and Modified Transudates

Protein concentrations less than 2.5–3.0 g/dL

Low nucleated cell count (<500–1000/µL)

Macrophages, lymphocytes, mesothelial cells

Right-sided heart failure, pericardial disease, hypoalbuminemia, neoplasia, diaphragmatic hernia

*Note:* Neoplastic cells may or may not be present in effusions caused by neoplastic processes.

## Eosinophilic Effusion

>10% of leukocytes are eosinophils

Reported in dogs in association with heartworm disease, systemic mastocytosis, interstitial pneumonia, and disseminated eosinophilic granulomatosis

## Thrombocyte Count

See Platelet Count

## Thyroid Function Tests

## Total $T_4$ (Thyroxine, Tetraiodothyronine)

Measures free $T_4$ and protein-bound $T_4$

Below-normal values suggest hypothyroidism (dogs).

Above-normal values in cats are likely caused by hyperthyroidism.

Below-normal values are also seen with underlying illness (sick, euthyroid).

## Free $T_4$ (f$T_4$)

Below-normal values suggest hypothyroidism (dogs).

Above-normal values in cats are likely caused by hyperthyroidism.

Not as affected by the suppressive effects of concurrent illness as total $T_4$

Modified equilibrium dialysis assay is not affected by circulating antithyroid hormone antibodies and therefore is the preferred assay for f$T_4$.

## Thyroid-Stimulating Hormone (TSH) Concentration

Must be interpreted in conjunction with serum $T_4$ and f$T_4$

Low value for serum $T_4$ and f$T_4$ with a high TSH supports diagnosis of hypothyroidism.

Normal $T_4$ and f$T_4$ and normal TSH rule out hypothyroidism.

## TSH and Thyroid-Releasing Hormone (TRH) Stimulation Tests

Used to differentiate hypothyroidism from euthyroid sick syndrome

These tests are not typically done because of availability and expense of reagents.

## $T_3$ (3,5,3'-Triiodothyronine) Concentration

Poor indicator of thyroid function in dogs and cats; not recommended

## Tests for Lymphocytic Thyroiditis

Autoantibodies to circulating thyroid hormone ($T_4$ and $T_3$) and thyroglobulin (Tg) correlate with lymphocytic thyroiditis.

Tg autoantibodies may be present when $T_4$ and $T_3$ are not; therefore testing for Tg autoantibodies is considered the better screening test.

Provides no information about the severity of disease or the extent of thyroid gland involvement

Hypothyroid dogs may be negative, and euthyroid dogs may have Tg autoantibodies.

May be used as a prebreeding screening test in breeding dogs

## $T_3$ Suppression Test

Administration of $T_3$ to normal cats should suppress pituitary TSH secretion, decreasing the serum $T_4$ concentration. Administration of $T_3$ to hyperthyroid cats should have no suppressive effect.

Confirms hyperthyroidism in cats with occult disease

## Toxoplasmosis Antibody Titer

Positive titer indicates exposure but not necessarily active infection.

Positive IgG with negative IgM titer is most consistent with chronic exposure.

Positive IgM titer greater than 1:256 is consistent with active infection, especially with typical clinical signs. Positive IgM titer with negative IgG titer may indicate recent infection.

Fourfold rise in IgG titer of paired samples 2–3 weeks apart also supports active infection.

## Triglycerides

*Normal Range*
Feline: 25–160 mg/dL
Canine: 29–291 mg/dL

*Elevated in:*
postprandial, familial triglyceridemia (Miniature Schnauzer, Beagle, other breeds); hyperchylomicronemia of cats (also observed in dogs); lipoprotein lipase deficiency (cat); endocrine disorders (hypothyroidism, hyperadrenocorticism, diabetes mellitus, acromegaly [cat]); nephrotic syndrome; pancreatitis; cholestasis; drugs (glucocorticoids, megestrol acetate)

*Decreased in:*
not clearly associated with any disease; severe malabsorptive protein-losing enteropathy, hyperthyroidism, chronic hepatopathies

## Trypsinogen-Like Immunoreactivity (TLI)

## Urinalysis

### Appearance

#### COLOR

*Yellow (normal):* may be dark amber when concentrated and pale to colorless when diluted. However, color does not always correlate with concentration.

*Red or reddish-brown*: hematuria, hemoglobinuria, myoglobinuria

*Dark brown or black*: methemoglobinuria

*Yellow-brown to yellow-green*: concentrated sample, bilirubinuria, *Pseudomonas* infection

*Orange*: bilirubinuria

#### TURBIDITY

Normally clear; cloudy urine may contain cellular material, crystals, lipid, and mucus

#### ODOR

Excess ammonia odor may be detectable in urine infected with urease-producing bacteria

## Urine Cortisol/Creatinine Ratio

Very sensitive but not very specific test for hyperadrenocorticism
Good test to rule out hyperadrenocorticism but not to diagnose

## Urine Protein/Creatinine Ratio

More accurate than dipstick protein estimation to assess for proteinuria
Normal values: dogs <0.3, cats <0.6

## von Willebrand Factor

Variable degrees of expression of factor for von Willebrand disease, a common, inherited hemostatic disorder (rare in cats)
Dogs with levels less than 30% are prone to spontaneous bleeding (e.g., epistaxis)
Classification of von Willebrand disease in dogs:
**Type I:** low concentration of normal von Willebrand factor
**Type II:** low-to-normal concentration of abnormal von Willebrand factor
**Type III:** absence of von Willebrand factor

Hemostatic screening tests usually are normal in dogs with von Willebrand disease

Buccal mucosal bleeding time is the exception—best screening test

## White Blood Cell Count

### Normal Range
Feline: 3.5–16.0×103/μL
Canine: 4.0–15.5×10³/μL

### Elevated in:
infection (bacterial, systemic mycoses); physiologic leukocytosis; metabolic (stress, glucocorticoids); inflammation (immune-mediated disease, neoplasia, tissue trauma, tissue necrosis); leukemia, associated with responsive anemia (hemorrhagic anemia, hemolytic anemia)

### Decreased in:
decreased production, increased consumption, neutropenia secondary to phenobarbital administration

# INDEX

Note: Page numbers followed by "*t*" indicate tables, and "*b*" indicate boxes.